Healing across Boundaries

This is a remarkable book on a remarkable topic. Optimal health of both the individual and the society is clearly dependent on contributions from a wide array of 'specialists', and Prof. Makarand Paranjape brings to us the views and opinions of not only distinguished medical practitioners and researchers, but also from luminaries in the field of psychology, philosophy, biology and social engineering. This stunning cast of contributors are responsible for the depth and breadth of topics covered, ranging from scientific temper to spirituality, from mind–body medicine to spiritual healing, from stress to *siddha*, and from ethics to economics. The book soars even higher by not trying to impose an unnatural harmony among the different viewpoints and come up with a common prescription. In an extremely endearing display of humility, the Editor aims to only provide a platform for a dialogue between practitioners on either side of the chasm. This book goes a long way in steering the debate from 'science versus spirituality' to 'science and spirituality'.

Dr A. J. Vinaya Simha
Professor of Endocrinology
Mayo Clinic, Rochester, Minnesota, USA

Healing across Boundaries

Bio-medicine and Alternative Therapeutics

Editor
Makarand R. Paranjape

Routledge
Taylor & Francis Group
LONDON AND NEW YORK

First published 2014 by Routledge

2 Park Square, Milton Park, Abingdon, Oxfordshire OX14 4RN
52 Vanderbilt Avenue, New York, NY 10017

Routledge is an imprint of the Taylor & Francis Group, an informa business

First issued in paperback 2019

Typeset by

Glyph Graphics Private Limited
23, Khosla Complex
Vasundhara Enclave
Delhi 110 096

British Library Cataloguing-in-Publication Data
A catalogue record of this book is available from the British Library

ISBN 978-1-138-79597-6 (hbk)
ISBN 978-0-367-17691-4 (pbk)

For Lalita,

hoping that she will contribute to the
art and science of healing across boundaries...

Contents

Foreword

Health in the 21st Century: Minding the Gap!

Over the last 150 years, bio-medical science has revolutionised our ability to recognise and combat disease, extending our life spans and maintaining fit and healthy lifestyles well into old age. The evidence is all around us. In the West, infections are not the threat they used to be. Smallpox, tuberculosis, syphilis, measles, diphtheria, typhoid, cholera, and poliomyelitis are rare, thanks largely to the combined efforts of public health and antibiotics. Duodenal ulcers are uncommon. Heart attacks can be prevented and treated rapidly. There are many effective treatments for cancer. As long as doctors can establish a pathological diagnosis, they can institute a cure, or at least an effective treatment. Yet, despite these impressive advances, more and more people in Western countries regard themselves as ill and are frustrated that the promise of modern scientific medicine does not seem to help them.

The spectacular advances in medical science have exposed a vast underbelly of illnesses for which there are no distinct causes and no specific treatments. The so-called 'medically unexplained illnesses', the diseases doctors cannot cure, afflict about 35 per cent of people attending community clinics and at least 50 per cent of those attending specialist services in hospitals. These ailments have names; people always find names for what they do not understand, usually calling them 'syndromes'. So, we have the chronic fatigue, irritable bowel, fibromyalgia, functional dyspepsia, and a myriad of other syndromes. But what is in a name — for 'unexplained illnesses' is merely an artifice by which doctors retain their threadbare mantle of control.

That is why I tend to make a distinction between diseases and illnesses. Diseases are objective, have well-defined pathologies, causes and specific treatments. Illnesses are subjective, related to what the patient experiences and therefore have much to do with diet, lifestyle and, more important than either of those, context and experience — what is happening in the patient's life. Diseases have mechanisms; illnesses have meaning. It is not always what is 'so' that makes us ill, but what we think is 'so'. That does not just involve the body, not even the mind and the body, but incorporates meaning as well. Mind, body and meaning; that, I would suggest, is the secular trinity of illness.

I prefer to use meaning in place of spirit or soul. In most Western countries, gone is the time when meaning inevitably led us to God, so the terms 'spirit' and 'soul' have lost the meaning they may once have had. What *is* spirituality, if not meaningfulness? When I am with a patient who has an unexplained illness, I listen with both my ears. My right ear is sifting the information, trying to catch any symptom or sign that might suggest specific pathology, while my left ear is listening to the story the patient is telling me and trying to discern connections — clues that explain what the illness means and how it expresses what cannot be talked about and needs to be 'brought to mind'.

But does that not underpin many traditional healing practices? First, understand your patient and then apply a 'meaningful' remedy that connects with their particular dynamic. That, as I see it, is the art of healing and, as such, needs a completely different mind-set to the science of medicine.

Nonetheless, in a properly integrated modern practice of medicine, the two must work together. Just as we use our two hands, two eyes, two ears, we also need to use both sides of our brain — our focused, analytic left brain and our integrative, narrative right brain — to understand and heal our patients. Practising one in preference to the other and the method will be lopsided and unbalanced and the patient will inevitably fall over.

Therefore, it is refreshing to read this illuminating series of essays by such diverse panel of scholars, doctors, scientists, philosophers and healers, who have 'dared to go where few have gone before'. This book moves us out of the safe prejudices of the 'mother ship' to explore the hinterlands between bio-medicine and healing, science and meaning, mechanism and narrative, and by doing so, attain an understanding of what it is to be ill.

But that is only one side of the equation. Getting well is not just something the healer does, it is what those who are unwell do. The role of healers is to use all the understanding and method at their disposal to assist the ailing to help themselves. Bio-medicine places too much emphasis on applying methods to make people well, and so, like an overindulgent parent, spoils the patient by failing to empower their own capacity for healing. Governments in the West have recently caught up with the traditional notion of empowering self-management for long-term illness, but one suspects they see this more as a way of saving money than as enlightened means of maintaining the health of the nation.

I sincerely hope that the scholarly essays and dialogues in this remarkable book will inspire medical students, doctors, healers of many disciplines, health managers and, above all, the billions of ailing people out there to help change their attitude. Healing and wellbeing is not just about mechanism, cause and cure, it is about meaning and narrative, and can only be effected by the ill person, guided and informed by healers with a sensitive understanding of both science and narrative, and the skill and intuition to 'bring out the best' in people.

Nick Read
Physician, Psychotherapist and Nutritionist
Formerly Professor of Physiology, University of Sheffield
Chair of the IBS Network — UK's national
charity for Irritable Bowel Syndrome

17 November 2013
Sheffield, UK

Preface

Modern medicine has made immense advances in both the technology and the effectiveness of healing. The result is that it has become the established medical practice of our world. While it has undoubtedly benefitted vast numbers of people, its hegemony has also limited other therapeutic methodologies and factors from playing a significant role in healing. Given the spiralling costs of providing healthcare today, modern bio-medicine has been criticised for being unethical and iniquitous. In addition, the medicalisation of life, the consideration of conditions not responding to bio-medicine as incurable, and the branding of other methods of engaging with illness as 'unscientific' pose serious challenges to its hegemony and effectiveness. While scientific progress continues to revolutionise medical care, innovative solutions have not always succeeded in preventing newer problems from surfacing. In a curious paradox, people in the developed world are turning in large numbers towards alternative systems of healthcare — labelled CAM or 'complementary and alternative medicine' — while those in developing countries have come under the increasing sway of modern bio-medicine.

Surveys have revealed that in the United States of America, the number of those seeking alternate therapeutics has been steadily rising in recent years. For instance, herbal supplements, energy medicine, prayer, bio-feedback, and massage have been gaining in popularity and acceptance. According to the National Center for Complementary and Alternative Medicine of the National Institute of Health of the United States, '[i]n 2007, almost 4 out of 10 adults had used CAM therapy in the past 12 months, with the most commonly used therapies being nonvitamin, nonmineral, natural products (17.7 per cent) and deep breathing exercises (12.7 per cent)' (Barnes et al. 2008: 1). In the fuller survey by the same organisation in 2002, the most common CAM therapies used in the USA in 2002 were prayer (45.2 per cent), herbalism (18.9 per cent), breathing meditation (11.6 per cent), meditation (7.6 per cent), chiropractic medicine (7.5 per cent), yoga (5.1 per cent), body work (5 per cent), diet-based therapy (3.5 per cent), progressive relaxation (3 per cent), mega-vitamin therapy (2.8 per cent), and visualisation (2.1 per cent) (Barnes et al. 2004). These trends in no way undermine the great progress that bio-medicine has made in modern times. They do, however, point to the limits of the bio-medical ideology to fully comprehend or explain the human situation in the context of health and disease. This state of affairs reflects fragmentation and incompleteness; it characterises a search for approaches that can complement and supplement standard bio-medical care and make it more wholesome.

The Indian scenario, interestingly, presents a striking contrast to the global situation. On the one hand, the prosperous elite reflects, at least superficially, the alternative-seeking behaviour characteristic of developed countries. On the other hand, India has of late witnessed a despiritualisation of its healing traditions, with the majority of the rural population being drawn to modern medical care. Even practitioners of traditional medical systems are often found prescribing allopathic medicines. Thus, in India we might notice the emergence of reductionism within the holistic framework of traditional medicine, while the global situation shows the emergence of holism within the reductionist framework of modern medicine.

While bio-medicine is thus gaining ground in India, it is not entirely certain whether it has been able to adapt itself to the Indian socio-cultural and economic realities. In that respect, the enabling structural factors for the emergence of bio-medicine as a well-established science are not uniformly present in India. Culturally, too, it remains largely disembedded and alien to Indian society. The large and glittering private hospitals in cities, which have made healthcare a ruthless business, seem like forbidding fortresses to the urban and rural under-classes. Given the existing scenario of widespread poverty and underdevelopment in India, perhaps bio-medicine needs to be more humane than professional, more integrated than specialised, more oriented to health than disease, more equitable than competitive, more community-oriented than market-driven. Many corrections have already been made in the dominant model of health and illness in Western countries, which are yet to be implemented in India.

That is why the stage appears set for alternative healthcare practices to provide a new framework that integrates psycho-spiritual approaches to healing with mainstream medical care. This is not essentially a picture of confrontation, but an awakening that recognises limitations, and harmonises the smaller with the bigger reality. It is not science *versus* spirituality, nor science *or* spirituality, but science *and* spirituality. For those who work outside the scientific paradigm, this is a most welcome change; both patients and practitioners are only too happy to discover supplementary paths to healing alongside the dominant medical approach. Cracks are beginning to appear on the hard walls of scientific authority, but many scientists are yet to be convinced. But surely, newer approaches to healing can also be subjected to scientific enquiry and scrutiny. The crux of the matter is how to impact what might be termed the trans-physical aspects of the human person, which demand as much attention as the body.

The time is ripe for a dialogue between the practitioners who stand on either side of the chasm. Medical traditions like Ayurveda, which are based on an integral understanding of the human person as a psycho-physical entity, have already worked out an approach to health and disease that combines science and spirituality as we understand the two today. In addition, other important medical systems like Siddha, homoeopathy, Tibetan medicine, and so on may be examined to glean a conceptual holistic framework in the context of healing.

This book is an attempt to open up this interesting and crucial field by crossing the boundaries between modern bio-medicine and traditional healing methods. It contains papers by medical doctors, bio-medical researchers, Ayurvedic practitioners, as well as philosophers, psychologists, sociologists, and cultural critics. No unified perspective is sought to be forced on the variety of views that are found here; the attempt, instead, is to problematise issues and encourage dialogue across disciplines. The contributors, as mentioned, are also from different walks of life, not all of them academics or social scientists, but also medical practitioners. There is thus not just disciplinary, but generic variety in the approaches and papers. The design of the volume is meant to show divergences and conflicts, as well as convergences and attempts at cooperation. As if to take our cue from Richard Rorty's post-epistemological method, we have tried to advance a 'conversationalist' view of knowledge, rather than a purely rationalist or empiricist position.

For instance, at the start of the book, in his conversation with the editor and Dr P. Ram Manohar, Professor Pushpa Bhargava, Founding Director, Centre for Cellular and Molecular Biology (CCMB), Hyderabad, one of India's most respected and recognised contemporary scientists, refuses to accept anything other or 'beyond' the natural or the physical, as might be expected of a trained and hardline modern biologist. He even considers the inquirer, that is, consciousness, to be reducible to brain functions. This provocative dialogue is succeeded by Ram Manohar's chapter, which takes a very different stance. As a certified Ayurvedic *vaidya* (doctor) and researcher, Ram Manohar's attempts to explicate the categories of 'science', 'spirituality', and 'healing' are enabling, in that they seek to make a dialogue across differing paradigms possible. As he shows, although less problematic than 'spirituality', the term 'science' also needs clearer definition when it comes to practical therapeutics. He observes how, in the Indian context, science and spirituality have at one point gone hand in hand. Ayurveda, the ancient and traditional art of healing in India, offers perhaps the best historical instance of how they were used together for human welfare. Ram Manohar looks at the continuing relevance of Ayurveda in today's world, dominated as it is by modern bio-medicine, also indicating how Ayurveda itself has changed with the altered context.

This introductory chapter is followed by individual interventions beginning with Dr Ramesh Bijlani's discussion of what lies beyond 'Mind–Body' medicine. Bijlani was Professor and Head of the Department of Physiology at the All India Institute of Medical Sciences (AIIMS), the leading national institution for research, teaching, and healthcare delivery in India. There he founded the Integral Health Clinic, and served as its director for several years. He argues that the power of the mind and body to heal itself is often unrecognised in clinical practice. In an alternative, more self-reliant approach to healing, this power becomes strengthened while lessening the habit of drug-dependence, which has become such an integral part of modern life. According to him, a healer can awaken the patient to the tremendous possibilities of self-healing, and help the patient use her/his own inner resources to harness these self-healing mechanisms. Furthermore, the living connection between the individual and the universe being can be used to channelise healing energies. The individual thus has an invisible but vital connection with the rest of creation. A healer can use this connection to lend a helping hand to the self-healing mechanisms of the patient. The chapter takes a closer look at viable alternatives to the methods of modern medicine, and provides certain instances where scientific medicine has now become open to accepting these possibilities.

The next chapter is by Dr O. P. Yadava, CEO and Chief Cardiac Surgeon at the National Heart Institute (NHI), New Delhi. Dr Yadava is also the editor-in-chief of *Cardiology Today* and *Annals of IMA Academy of Medical Specialities*. He probes into the role spirituality plays not just in healing specific diseases, but in the overall wellness of a person. If healing stands for more than just the physical amelioration of disease, then its primary concern is the restoration of all-round wellbeing or wholeness in an individual. In such a process, spirituality becomes an indispensible part. He asks how personal beliefs affect a patient, and how faith impacts disease. According to him, a patient's beliefs and faith may influence recovery psychologically, but more importantly, also affect coping and end-of-life issues. Since religion and spirituality are inexorably linked with the concept of illness, especially in a country like India, faith comes to play a major part in the patient's experiential encounter with illness and the possibility of death. Therefore, faith and spirituality can become important allies to induce healing in an ailing subject. It is a known fact today that the stress of the modern lifestyle is the rootcause of many cardiovascular ailments and imbalances in neuro-hormonal levels, blood pressure, and heart rate. Simpler and cheaper therapies, such as meditation, rhythmic breathing exercises and a spiritual lifestyle, which combat negative stress without the use of invasive surgery or multiple pharmacotherapy, may go a long way in reducing the incidence of heart disorders. They have even more relevance in developing and financially impoverished countries like India, where alternative medicine may help many without the debilitating physical and financial consequences of expensive medicinal and surgical procedures. This chapter also makes a case for the benefits that may accrue from a coalition of alternative and the more accepted, current bio-medical clinical medical practices.

The author of Chapter Four, 'Healing Minds and Bodies: What Place for Spirituality?' Professor Roger Worthington is a philosopher by training, responsible for teaching medical law and ethics at Keele University School of Medicine. He takes a closer look at the relationship between the healer and the healed from the standpoint of Indian spirituality, especially the Himalayan traditions of Saiva Siddhanta in their exploration of consciousness. In line with the suggestions mooted by the earlier chapters, he too believes that minds and bodies are part of an integrated whole; if bodies do not heal in the way that they should, there may be extra-physical explanations for why this is so. One of these might be that the underlying causes are reflective of a disturbed state of mind, and lack of equilibrium or wellbeing. By this account, if self-alienation or the break in union is the root cause of illness, then questions arise as to what the best remedies to try and restore wholeness are. This chapter looks for answers by exploring the relationships between 'healer', 'healing', and 'the healed' within a broad context of science and spiritual philosophy. The practice of medicine is a shared enterprise in which physician and patient both play a role. If one believes that there is a spiritual dimension to healing, then bio-medicine and spiritual healing can reasonably co-exist, and if that position is accepted, the apparent dichotomy between scientific and spiritual explanations for healing becomes redundant. The brain may indeed be bound to the body, but the mind is universal, and this chapter is a discussion of the mind's power of healing, with particular reference to Indian traditions of spirituality and self-discipline.

Chapter Five, 'The Culture and Philosophy of Bio-medicine in India', is by a sociologist, Professor Suhita Chopra Chatterjee, who teaches at the Indian Institute of Technology, Kharagpur (IIT-K). She critiques the prevalent culture and philosophy of bio-medicine in India in the light of the current understanding of its features in the West. What are the social and cultural implications of the globalisation of bio-medicine, which began as a distinctly Western system of healing? When it is researched and practised in a variety of cultural contexts, how does modern bio-medicine need to change or adapt itself? According to her, the bio-medical view of the human being and of human suffering is too body-centric and reductive. She is also concerned with issues of equity and access, especially in a poorer country like India. Her plea is that rather than seeing it as a single, unitary entity, bio-medicine may be viewed as a plurality of practices that need to be socially and culturally situated. Otherwise, its built-in insensitivity to and intolerance of plural healthcare systems will only endanger traditional medical practices like Ayurveda, which have served the common people for so many centuries.

In Chapter Six, 'Spirituality, Mental Health, and Perfectionism', Dr Nilanjana Sanyal, Professor of Clinical and Developmental Psychology at University of Calcutta, examines the issue of mental health in the light of research on 'perfectionism'. The author uses the term 'psychological wealth' to denote a holistic sense of physical and emotional wellbeing. Psychological wealth means finding satisfaction in daily human experiences, realising the self through the pursuit of important goals, and the achievement of positive emotions through their accomplishment. The drive to 'perfection', when excessive, may prove detrimental to such wellness, even leading to pathological maladjustment and depression. Instead, more realistic goals, tempered by an acceptance of the subject's limitations, may lead to a more balanced life. To her, the inter-relatedness of the mind and the body, which psychologists have studied extensively, is the key to health. It is often observed that many physical ailments have their roots in the mind, and in the mind also lies the power to heal them. This chapter turns to the mind or the psyche, and the importance of its wellbeing in order to live a truly healthy life. Our psyche dictates much of how and what we experience in life; ultimately, it becomes the root cause of health or the absence of it. In this context, the practice of spirituality becomes an important part of building positive emotions. In a materialistic world, success and perfectionism become obsessions which often lead to an unfulfilled, anxious existence. It is of utmost importance, then, to build a culture of positive living, which can then bring about psychological growth not only in adults, but also in children who emulate the former. Since most of our ailments today point towards various psychological maladjustments that we carry from our early childhoods, the creation of a positive emotional atmosphere for young children and adolescents must become a priority. An excessive drive towards perfection may cause many imbalances and illnesses. From the point of view of clinical psychology, which relies heavily on the mind–body connections and their implications, this chapter charts the connections between psychological health and spirituality, and how together they can create a truly healthy subject.

Chapter Seven, 'The Doctrine of the Three Humours in Traditional Indian Medicine' by noted Indologist Hartmut Scharfe is a valuable contribution not only to our understanding of Ayurveda, but also to its relationship with the Siddha tradition in Tamil Nadu. The idea of the three *dosa*s also finds its parallels in the medical theory based on humours widely prevalent in pre-modern Europe. Scharfe, tracing the textual roots of this idea in ancient Tamil texts finds that it does not have pre-Ayurvedic antecedents. This leads him to argue that the latter must have influenced the former. Scharfe asks the key questions: how old is Siddha medicine and how does it relate to the better known Ayurveda, since both have much in common and are practised side by side in south India? Confronted with conflicting claims put forth with equal vehemence, Scharfe offers a balanced and plausible perspective, especially considering how ideologically embroiled such issues have become.

In Chapter Eight, 'The Body in the System of Medicine: Caraka and Harvey', Dr Anuradha Veeravalli, who teaches Philosophy at the University of Delhi, compares the theoretical presupposes of traditional and alternative healing systems like Ayurveda and those of modern clinical medicine. One of the main differences between them is that modern bio-medicine relies on empirical, physical evidence, while the earlier systems depended on 'natural philosophy'. The chapter analyses the significance of the discussion on *sarirasthanam* (the foundation of the body) in the *Carakasamhita* in relation to the principles of the new post-Enlightenment system of medicine, which came to be established with the publication in 1628 of William Harvey's *The Circulation of the Blood*. The latter decisively established the effectiveness of the principles of the scientific method, that is, experiment and analysis, in new science for modern times. Harvey consciously denied any association with philosophy, as did his contemporaries, who argued that anatomy, and not philosophy, was the basis of medicine. The *Sarirasthanam* section in the *Carakasamhita* presents a particularly interesting study of the relation between science and religion since it disallows the separation of the two disciplines, again much to the discomfort of both the spiritualist and the scientist. The body as the object of study of the theory of longevity is the seat of the union of self/spirit and matter. Caraka argues that the sense organs that make possible the experience of pain and pleasure, and of life and death, are proof of this fact, because mere matter can feel no pain. It is only matter animated by the spirit that makes for sentient beings. If healing deals with such beings, then it must include the spirit in some form. The chapter concludes with a discussion of the idea of the body in Mahatma Gandhi's conception of 'Nature Cure', and in the scheme of organic living as envisioned by his philosophy.

The next chapter is 'Network of Touch in Spiritual Healing: *Pancikarana-prakriya*', by Dr Piyali Palit, Professor of Philosophy at Jadavpur University, who is also trained in classical Sanskrit. She explores how the notion of *pancikarana*, or the network of five elements spoken of in ancient scriptures, may contribute to healing. The basic five elements referred to in such texts are created in a chain from the *Atman* — the real nature of each and every being — to the outermost sense organs. But this *Atman* is itself devoid of the physique and therefore, in the *Atman* resides eternal bliss, associated with eternal consciousness and perennial existence. Human beings, on the contrary, are captured by six types of *vikaaras* (changes), and are continuously going through *duhkha* or suffering that originates from their own actions. To reconcile this apparent contradiction between our daily experience of mutability and our ultimate reality as changeless selves, she resorts to Vaisesika formal ontology to suggest that the *Atman* extends itself through a network of elements in a systematic pervasion. In this network, touch plays a very important role because living creatures react to it right from their birth, even before they have visual sensation. In the process of spiritual healing, the impurities in the body are supposed to be eliminated and/or replaced by pure elements. Therefore, healing through touch involves the transference of sensation from the physical to the *antahkarana* or the mind, which in turn transfers that sensation to the *Atman*, thus bringing the tangible and the intangible together.

Carrying on the analysis of traditional texts, Dr Asha Mukherjee, Professor of Philosophy at Visva-Bharati, Santiniketan, turns her attention to 'Bio-ethical Issues: Jaina Perspective and Prospects'. This chapter discusses some important medical-ethical issues from the framework of Jainism, a major religious tradition that puts *ahimsa* or non-violence at the heart of its practice. How does it react to modern bio-medicine, which is based on the vivisection of and experimentation on animals? The deep interconnection between health, life and death, and how religion influences them, becomes once again a crucial point of discussion in this chapter. What may be observed in this regard is that Jaina practice has not remained static. On the contrary, under the impact of modernity in general and bio-medicine more specifically, we see the emergence of a modern ethical discourse within and for a Jaina laity, whose concerns throughout history have generally been more diverse and variable than those of the ascetic community. Some of the latter, following the tenets of their faith rigorously, would find bio-medicine totally unethical, while the former have evolved means of co-existing with, and even resorting to, it.

In Chapter Eleven, '"Yogi-doctors" and Occult Healing Arts: Holistic Therapeutics at Sri Aurobindo Ashram', I document a significant therapeutic practice reported from the Sri Aurobindo Ashram, Pondicherry, during its formative years from the 1930s to the 1960s. The Ashram was then presided over by its masters, first Sri Aurobindo (1872–1950) and Mira Richard or the Mother (1878–1973) together, and then, after the death of the former in 1950, by the latter. Although the worldview embodied in this practice belongs to a modern, even futuristic, spiritual movement, yet the 'knowledge' on health and healing used by its members bears a close resemblance not only to submerged and occult traditions in both the East and the West, but also to the main indigenous system of healthcare in India, namely

Ayurveda. In addition, this chapter is distinctly 'post-colonial' in its interpretation of a rich archive of narratives, and thus the textuality of healing practices. In other words, it is about 'stories' of healing and how we read them, and not just about the substance of the stories. In this case, the 'narrativity' of these healing practices is read in terms of their power relations to dominant bio-medical therapeutics, and the now subaltern indigenous systems. In that sense, the Aurobindonian system represents alternative paradigms of knowledge or contending epistemologies. That is why its healing stories may be read as examples of 'insurgent knowledges', or what Michel Foucault called the 'insurrection of subjugated knowledges'. Interestingly, these 'insurgent knowledges' were resurrected, enunciated, further developed, and propped up by the personal authority of the Gurus. Eventually, such healing knowledges became part of a 'magico-religious system' centred on the vast output of the Gurus, studied and perpetuated by the Ashram community.

The volume concludes with a multi-participant discussion on 'The Science and Spirituality of Healing', originally recorded before a live audience in the studios of Amrita Viswavidyalaya. The panelists and speakers include: Dr O. P. Yadava (CEO and Chief Cardiac Surgeon, NHI, New Delhi), Shri Michel Danino (Convenor for the International Forum for India's Heritage), Vaidya Dr P. Ram Manohar (Director of Research at the Arya Vaidya Pharmacy, Coimbatore), Dr Ramesh Bijlani (Aurobindo Ashram, New Delhi), Dr Nisha Money (United States Air Force and the University of Health Sciences, Preventive Medicine and Biometrics, USA), Dr Matthew Fritts (Clinical Research Associate, Samueli Institute, Virginia, USA), Tom McKenzie (Global Perspectives on Science and Spirituality), Dr V. Sujatha (Associate Professor at the Centre for Study of Social Systems, Jawaharlal Nehru University), and Dr Rama Jayasundar (AIIMS, New Delhi). Addressing various issues and implications of 'science' as a category with enforceable boundaries, the discussion focuses on the possibilities and pitfalls in trying to integrate modern bio-medicine and alternative healing practices. Recognised medical practitioners, one from AIIMS, and the other from the NHI, both of whom set great store by the benefits of alternate and spiritual healing practices, thus interact with philosophers, psychologists, sociologists of medicine, and cultural critics from reputed institutions such as IIT-K, Jadavpur University, Calcutta University, Visva-Bharati, University of Delhi, and Jawaharlal

Nehru University. This concluding section thus consists of a lively and wide-ranging symposium in which the different views presented are brought into sharper relief, and possibilities of co-existence, if not integration, are explored.

Most of the chapters in this volume are revised papers first presented at a conference on 'Science and Spirituality in Healing', held near Coimbatore, south India, from 15–17 January 2008. The conference was a collaborative venture between the project on 'Indian Perspectives on Science and Spirituality' of the Jawaharlal Nehru University, New Delhi, and the Ayurvedic Research wing of the Arya Vaidya Pharmacy (Coimbatore), one of the largest providers of Ayurvedic healthcare in India. The main thrust of both the conference and this book is to explore if and how healing, as a process, appears to involve both the physical and what may be termed the trans-physical dimensions of being. As such, Ayurveda, among other traditional medical systems such as Siddha, Unani, and Tibetan medicine, already presupposes such a unity of the physical and the trans-physical. Allopathy or modern medicine, on the other hand, until recently seemed to embody a split between the 'scientific', that is, physical, and the trans-physical, that is, the 'spiritual' dimensions of healing. How may these apparently incommensurable views be brought to a face-off, if not a dialogue? This is the central question of the volume.

With growing affluence and longevity, health and wellness have become multi-billion dollar industries worldwide. There are numerous books on alternative healing practices, apart from thousands devoted to self-help and inspirational self-improvement. However, this volume embodies a rare coming together on the same platform of practitioners of modern bio-medicine, Ayurvedic and alternate healers, philosophers and sociologists of healing, as well as cultural theorists and historians, in an attempt to understand the complex and boundary-crossing nature of healing. I hope that it will generate an active and lively interest across the spectrum of practitioners of healing arts, both modern and traditional, as well as those interested in wellbeing and integral medicine.

Before closing, I might hazard a definition of 'spirituality', at least as it has been used in this volume. It is no doubt a word with fuzzy connotations and boundaries, which suggests a variety of meanings, ranging from 'the state or quality of being dedicated to God, religion, or spiritual things or values', 'the condition or quality of being spiritual', 'a distinctive approach to religion or prayer', to 'Church property or revenue or a Church benefice' (www.dictionary.com). As far as this book is concerned, none of these definitions is actually apt, although the common element running through them perhaps is. This common element is the notion that 'spiritual' refers to the non-material or non-corporeal part of our being. In medieval times, such a distinction between body and soul was widely accepted. Even today, a vast number of human beings all over the world regard themselves as not just their bodies. Among the Judeo-Christian traditions, the idea of the soul is a cardinal belief, as it was among the Greeks and Egyptians before them (see, for instance, McGraw 2004).

Most Hindus also accept the idea of the 'Atman' or a divine element as constituting their real self. Buddhists, Taoists, animists, pantheists, and many others also have some idea of an extra-physical dimension to the individual. Buddhism, for instance, although it does not recognise a permanent, unchanging self, is not immaterialist; rather, it identifies many subtle layers of the mind and mental processes that are different from and can affect the body. Modern science, of course, does not accept, at least officially, the existence of any such entity as soul or spirit, but it does understand mind, psyche, or consciousness to be a special aspect or feature of bodily existence. To us, all these trans-physical or supra-corporeal aspects may be taken as constituting the domain of healing practices that try to go beyond the body. The chapters in this volume discuss various aspects of such an idea of 'spirituality', including psychology, mind–body healing, yoga, meditation, and other spiritual practices, the reduction of stress as a way to prevent disease, and also bigger issues such as the relation of the individual to God, universe, or some other bigger entity or power, a belief in which may affect the process of healing. What is more, it also looks at spirituality in terms of holistic or integrative therapeutic practices such as Ayurveda or Siddha, in comparison with the largely body-centric and mechanistic ideology of modern bio-medicine. Needless to say, our intention here is not to preach or recommend any particular position, but to hear different voices and examine the possibilities of dialogue.

A project of this sort would not have come to the publication stage without the help and support of a large number of people. My thanks, first of all, to Global Perspectives on Science and Spirituality (GPSS), led by Professor Pranab Das and Tom Mackenzie, who funded it. Tom himself came to the conference and took part in the deliberations.

Arya Vaidya Pharmacy led by Shri P. R. Krishnakumar, a dynamic visionary leader in the field of Ayurveda, provided not only local support, but Dr P. Ram Manohar of the Aarya Vaidya Trust Institute of Advanced Research (AVTAR) collaborated at every stage. The venue of the conference was the Arsha Vidya Gurukulam, an advanced centre for the study and teaching of Vedanta, located at picturesque Anaikatti in the Nilgiri hills, near Coimbatore. My thanks to Swami Dayananda Saraswati, the founder and head, for hosting us, and also for presiding over the inaugural session. I am grateful to all the participants, especially those who contributed papers — the medical doctors, Ayurvedic vaidyas, practitioners of Siddha and Tibetan medicine, and academics from the diverse range of disciplines. The Project Cell of the Jawaharlal Nehru University, as well as my project assistants, helped throughout, as did my colleagues at the Centre for English Studies, who did not frown upon one of their own going a bit too far from the Centre's main concerns. I am also grateful to the Centre's UGC Special Assistance Programme for supporting the publication of this volume. My special thanks to my student Prayag Ray for his meticulous editorial assistance. Finally, kudos to the team at Routledge, India, for their faith in this volume and unfailing guidance in seeing it into print.

References

Barnes, P. M., B. Bloom and R. Nahin. 2008. 'Complementary and Alternative Medicine Use Among Adults and Children: United States, 2007', *CDC National Health Statistics Report*, 12: 1–23.

Barnes, P., E. Powell-Griner, K. McFann, and R. Nahin. 2004. 'Complementary and Alternative Medicine Use Among Adults: United States, 2002', *CDC Advance Data Report*, 343.

McGraw, John J. 2004. *Brain & Belief: An Exploration of the Human Soul.* Del Mar, CA: Aegis Press.

Rorty, Richard. 1998. *Truth and Progress: Philosophical Papers*, Vol. 3.Cambridge: Cambridge University Press.

Introduction: The Terms of the Dialogue

*A Conversation with Pushpa Mittra Bhargava and P. Ram Manohar**

Makarand R. Paranjape

Professor Makarand R. Paranjape (henceforth **MRP**): Thank you, Professor Bhargava and Dr Ram Manohar for the privilege of having this conversation on 'the science and spirituality of healing'. This exchange is significant not only because both of you are eminent professionals in the field, but also because you represent two different approaches to healing. Dr Bhargava, in addition to being the founding Director of the Centre for Cellular and Molecular Biology (Hyderabad), you are one of India's most eminent biologists, with an abiding interest in public health. You, Dr Ram Manohar, besides being a trained Ayurvedic *vaidya* (doctor), are one of our most eminent researchers in the field, having conducted several studies and clinical trials on Ayurvedic medicine. I am grateful to you both for this opportunity to converse on a subject that is of interest to a growing number of people, both healthcare givers and recipients.

Professor Pushpa Mittra Bhargava (henceforth **PMB**): Perhaps, before we start, I should confess that one major problem I have is that we rarely find a clear definition of spirituality, unlike science, which is clearly well defined. For example, does the concept of spirituality involve the existence of the supernatural, which would be outside the scope of science?

MRP: In our theme note on this topic, we defined spirituality as the trans-physical aspects of the human person, which, it is increasingly acknowledged, demand as much attention as does the body. Further, we wished to ask if the stage appears set for alternative healthcare practices to provide a new framework that integrates psycho-spiritual approaches to healing with mainstream medical care.

PMB: I take it that by 'trans-physical aspects of the human person', you mean aspects that are outside of the scope of science. I am afraid there is no aspect of the human being — or for that matter, of life in any form — that is outside of the scope of science. There is not a shred of evidence in favour of the existence of the soul or spirit. For every phenomenon concerning living systems (including consciousness and free will), there are either already established scientific explanations, or there are valid reasons to believe that such explanations will be found.

Dr P. Ram Manohar (henceforth **PRM**): But what is the soul or spirit being denied here? We need clear definitions. Can we deny the consciousness that makes this discussion possible? It is awareness itself that is the ultimate proof of science. No science would be possible without consciousness. We cannot deny the tongue with the tongue. Most of the popular notions of soul and spirit will not stand the test of Vedantic enquiry. There are rational explanations of the self, which need to be studied and differentiated from simplistic or 'unscientific' notions.

MRP: More specifically, we noted that Complimentary or Alternative Medicine (CAM) is finding increasing acceptance in the West. This includes herbal supplements, yoga, energy medicine, prayer, biofeedback, massage, and so on. For instance, in 2007, almost four out of 10 adults had used CAM therapy in the past 12 months, with the most commonly used therapies being nonvitamin, nonmineral, natural products (17.7 per cent) and deep breathing exercises (12.7 per cent). American Indian or Alaska Native adults (50.3 per cent) and white adults (43.1 per cent) were more likely to use CAM than Asian adults (39.9 per cent) or black adults (25.5 per cent). Between 2002 and 2007, increased use was seen among adults for acupuncture, deep breathing exercises, massage therapy, meditation, naturopathy, and yoga. Prayer has not been included in the survey.

PMB: What happens in the West does not automatically become rational. For example, was the US invasion of Vietnam, Iraq or Afghanistan, or support to Islamic fundamentalism and terrorism in the beginning rational?

PRM: Just as what happens in the West does not automatically become rational, what happens in India does not automatically become irrational either.

MRP: We are well aware that spirituality is a fuzzy area when it comes to clear-cut definitions. At the most basic, it implies a non-corporeal element to the human person, what some have called soul, spirit, self, or consciousness. At the other extreme, many hold that spirit is everything because matter, too, is nothing but spirit.

At this juncture, may I also submit that what is meant by 'science' is not wholly clear either. Originally, the word simply meant 'knowledge'. Modern science was called natural philosophy before the scientific method set itself up as the only reliable means of verifiable knowledge.

Even in the domain of science, what Kuhn calls 'paradigm shifts' fundamentally affect what is considered valid.

Most scientists would agree that what we call science today is only the name given to a particular methodology or epistemology. Not everything is amenable to it as yet. Yet, several scientists would have an objection to our definition of 'trans-physical' for spiritual aspects of healing. For them, everything, including consciousness, mind, or self, would be ultimately reducible to some physical or material object.

PMB: What is meant by science is, I believe, not fuzzy. The characteristics of the method of science and the attributes of knowledge gained through this method have no ambiguity (see Bhargava and Chakrabarti 2007). The paradigm shifts in science mentioned by Kuhn are always within the framework defined earlier.

PRM: Science has indeed been more clearly defined than religion or spirituality, and it is true that several religious or spiritual belief systems and science are incompatible. But systems like Ayurveda are not belief systems and are not based on unquestionable dogmas. They are dogmatic only to the extent that science has also become dogmatic in practice, in the hands of vested interests.

MRP: But don't you think that the very distinction between natural and supernatural needs to be problematised?

PMB: I don't see any problem in distinguishing between the natural and the supernatural. The former comes within the purview of science. The latter is outside of the scope of science. Science, by definition, does not accept the existence of the supernatural, for which there is no evidence whatsoever. Therefore, if you make today a survey of, say, the Nobel Prize winners in science after 1950, the Fellows of the Royal Society of London, and members of other major national science academies in the West, you would probably find that well over 95 per cent are non-believers. Indeed, there is an inherent incompatibility between science on the one hand, and religious beliefs or dogma on the other.

PRM: But don't you think that science has become such an established religion that even Nobel laureates are conformists?

MRP: Also, everything outside the present purview of science may not be non-existent or unreal. Conversely, why people adhere to 'beliefs and dogmas' themselves may have a 'scientific' explanation some day. But let us move on, rather than getting bogged down with difficulties in 'naming'.

Let me ask you a more specific question: In the context of your views on the health care scenario in 2050, what place do you envisage for CAM?

PMB: Out of the present repertoire of CAM systems and treatments, only two — properly validated and standardised plant-based drug formulations, and physiotherapeutic systems such as yoga — are likely to be a part of the healthcare scenario in 2050.

PRM: The latest statistics on the usage of CAM in the US reveals that meditation and deep breathing figure amongst the most widely used CAM interventions. Also, CAM has inspired a new approach to medicine called integrative medicine, which aims to look at the body, mind and self of the human person. CAM approaches are being integrated with conventional medicine to make it more holistic and sensitive to the dimensions of the mind and self.

MRP: Ayurveda is thought to be a holistic system of treatment, in that it addresses not only symptoms, but also the underlying causes of disease. What is more, like other holistic systems such as yoga or Tantra, it integrates lifestyle, ethics and worship in the healing process. To what extent do you think this a valid approach? Should our focus merely be on curing disease or on all-round wellbeing?

PMB: The focus in the modern systems of medicine is both on curing disease and on all-round wellbeing. It is a mistake to believe that Ayurveda addresses the underlying causes of disease and is a holistic system. For example, does Ayurveda tell us the underlying cause of hepatitis, AIDS, stomach ulcers, small pox, or malaria? It is modern medicine that demands that we understand and address the underlying cause of disease. Modern medicine is, in fact, truly holistic and places great emphasis on lifestyle in every disease — be it diabetes or cardiac disorders. The Hippocratic oath, subsequent declarations like the Helsinki Declaration, and a host of other stipulations such as stringent requirements for clinical trials, are an integral part of the ethics of the practice of modern medicine. It is not the fault of the system that there is corruption and lack of ethics in practice. This corruption exists everywhere, including CAM. Tantra, worship, and systems like homeopathy or witchcraft are nothing short of absurd; whatever apparently good effect they have is like that of a placebo. Modern medicine is concerned both with curing disease and all-round wellbeing in a far more scientific and effective way than CAM, which almost always invokes mumbo-jumbo.

PRM: Ayurveda does not claim to understand everything about diseases. There are certain advantages in the Ayurvedic approach to understanding diseases, and there are disadvantages too. Ayurveda is all about facilitating healing; it is essentially not about understanding every detail of a disease. When Ayurveda talks about underlying causes, it means conditions in the body that make the body vulnerable to disease, and not the instrumental causes (*nimitta karana*) that have been the focus in modern medicine. There are fundamental differences in the way disease causation is interpreted in both systems. Ayurveda lays great emphasis on individual variations in response to diseases, personalisation of treatment, mind–body interactions, and immunological responses. It is a dictum in Ayurveda that treatment should be a combination of medicine (*aushadha*), diet (*ahara*), and lifestyle modification (*vihara*).

Also, it is a sweeping statement that modern medicine is truly holistic; it ignores the dark side of modern medicine. The reductionist approach of modern medicine has been well-documented and critiqued by eminent scientists. While it is a fact that modern medicine is beginning to understand the role of lifestyle in a few diseases like diabetes and heart disease, there is not enough evidence to believe that it has elaborated truly holistic and lifestyle-based interventions for every disease.

As for mumbo-jumbo, CAM invokes mumbo-jumbo to the extent that pharmaceutical giants are compromising the quality of medical research and releasing unethical and dangerous drugs for human use from time to time. We cannot shut our eyes and ears to the mumbo-jumbo that is being propagated in the name of science either. Not only modern medicine, but every human initiative has also been maligned by corruption and lack of ethics in practice. Ayurveda cannot be blamed either if its practice has been affected by corruption and malpractices in the course of its evolution. Some of the most brilliant Western scholars on the history of medicine have paid glowing tributes to the high ethical standards outlined in the Ayurvedic texts. Karin Preisendanz, a noted scholar of Nyaya from Vienna, referred to a passage in the *Caraka Samhita* as the 'speech of initiation', and pointed out the inappropriateness of making loose correlations with the Greek tradition, as many scholars have done before. Labelling this passage the 'Hippocratic oath' in Ayurvedic texts is to impose Western notions on the latter. How many Indians know that *Caraka Samhita* was the first textbook on medicine to differentiate between accidental clinical outcomes and those responsive to treatment? Caraka says that if you cannot substantiate a successful clinical outcome with evidence, then it should be dismissed as having been caused by chance.

Caraka Samhita also differentiates between diseases that are self-limiting, diseases that are reversible by active treatment, and diseases that do not respond to treatment. Caraka warns the physician that it is foolish to make claims of having treated self-limiting diseases. Some of the earliest Ayurvedic texts distinguish between a true drug response (*nirmantra*) and the so-called placebo effect (*samantra*). However, Ayurveda encourages the invoking of the placebo effect in treatment. Even a practitioner of modern medicine cannot escape creating a placebo effect in the process of healing. The placebo effect is inapplicable only in clinical trials, not in clinical practice. There is no denying the limited applicability of using placebos in research. Not employing the placebo effect in clinical practice is to kill the initiative of the mind to trigger the process of healing. We are mental beings as much as we are physical beings and as long as the mind is active, the placebo effect will manifest. Ayurveda thinks that every clinical outcome is a combination of the placebo effect and the drug effect. We will have to become machines to completely transcend the placebo effect. If a clinician asserts that the placebo effect does not manifest in the actual practice of modern medicine, he is treating machines and not human beings. In order to validate a causal relationship between events, the ancient texts talk about using three arms — *paksha* (the context where a causal relationship is suspected, for example, a trial drug); *sapaksha* (the context where a causal relationship is already established, for example, a control drug); and *vipaksha* (the context where a causal relationship is proved to be non-existent, for example, placebo). There are many more examples of contrivances that were used to validate knowledge and differentiate it from mere beliefs.

MRP: With contrasting epistemologies, do you think it is possible to integrate modern and traditional medical systems?

PMB: Only to the extent mentioned earlier, minus religious mumbo-jumbo.

PRM: Opinion varies among scientists on the issue of integration, depending on their exposure to traditional medical systems and the effort put in to study them dispassionately. I believe that what will ultimately survive the test of time is truth minus not only religious mumbo-jumbo, but also 'scientific' mumbo-jumbo. Science is as prone as religion to propagate the mumbo-jumbo that misleads human minds. Neither has science escaped the evils of institutionalisation and power politics.

MRP: In your own tenure as Director, CCMB, you took an initiative to acquire the work of some of our leading contemporary painters. To what extent do you think that aesthetics or the quest for, and appreciation of, beauty could be one common pursuit in both science and culture?

PMB: Both science and art are committed to beauty and have a very strong relationship. Aesthetic appreciation is almost certainly built in our genes. In fact, science and art are two sides of the same coin. A great deal of work has been done on how our brain responds to good music, painting and sculpture.

MRP: While it is clear that science fosters a certain culture, notably of rationality and progress, to what extent do you think that it is itself a product of culture?

PMB: Science is a product of man's innate curiosity, rationality and ability to ask questions. Those societies or cultures which have recognised this and supported questioning have had much greater chances of flourishing on a continuing basis. Thus, while scientific truths are culture- and value-free, culture does influence the quality and quantity of the science done. In fact, in today's world, the greatest impediment to science is religious dogma and dictatorship of any kind.

PRM: I agree that the greatest impediment to science and knowledge is dogma of any kind. In fact, the greatest appeal of Indian culture is its rational approach and its support of questioning.

MRP: Would you say that Indian traditions give us a totally different perspective on issues such as evolution or even cloning? While the former is still contentious in the US, even when Darwin's book was first published, it did not cause any ripples in India. Some Swamijis have told me that that is because Hindus always accept evolution as a principle. The concept of the *Dashavatars*, for instance, indicates a gradual ascent from lower forms of life to full-fledged human, and then suprahuman beings. As to cloning, our mythology not only has similar ideas, but since the body is regarded as merely a vehicle, there is no great anxiety about what would happen if cloning human beings were legalised. The Dalai Lama, for instance, when asked about this said that as long as what we produce is a sentient being, it will be equally in need of compassion as other sentient beings. Professor Narlikar said to me that the idea of the Big Bang is very Judeo-Christian because it mirrors creationist notions, while that of the expanding and contracting, but always existing, universe is closer to Eastern ideas. Once again, do you think cultural issues affect the outcome of science?

PMB: The concept of 'evolution', such as the *Dashavatars*, which you have attributed to Hinduism, has nothing to do with Darwinian evolution. Our ancestors (for that matter, no one till Darwin talked about it) knew nothing about Darwinian evolution. Linnaeus and Wallace came closest, but that was about the time of Darwin. Darwin's *Origin of Species* did not cause a ripple in India when it was published, 150 years ago, because India was in the scientific backwaters of the world. Modern scicncc had taken root and flourished in Europe after the Renaissance, which never happened in India — except possibly in Bengal to a limited extent in the late 19th and early 20th century.

The view of a large section of the American population on evolution and its support to creationism is surely an expression of its intellectual backwardness and lack of knowledge — reminiscent of what the Church did to Copernicus, Galileo and Bruno. There is no tradition in India of understanding either evolution or cloning — neither from the point of view of the science involved in it, nor its consequences. I don't believe the Dalai Lama understands cloning or its consequences. For example, there are two types of cloning, therapeutic and reproductive. By and large, in the civilised world (excepting in the US, till at least recently) there has been no problem with therapeutic cloning. Reproductive cloning makes no sense, as an individual is a product of both genetics and environment. To consider the human body merely a vehicle for something such as an immortal soul is, in the light of today's knowledge, nothing short of charlatanism. We must learn to let ideas such as that of soul or spirit die a natural death.

As regards Jayant Narlikar, whom I have known well for four decades, he was one of the co-authors of the theory of the expanding and contracting, but always existing, universe. I do not bclievc that the now widely accepted idea of the Big Bang mirrors creationist notions. It actively mirrors more the evolutionary notions, as 10^{-41} or 10^{-42} seconds after the Big Bang, we had, successively, physical evolution, astrophysical evolution, chemical evolution, and biological evolution.

As I have already said, cultural ideas (specifically religious ideas) surely affect (adversely) the practice of science, and therefore its outcome in society. Example: the Islamic world.

PRM: Darwin's theory of evolution cannot be compared with the *Dashavatar*. The *Dashavatar* is all about psycho-spiritual evolution and not just the origin of species. The *Dashavatar* is not antagonistic to Darwin's theory, however. While many notions in Hindu scriptures do contradict the views in the Bible, a closer study of biblical accounts of creation and accounts of creation in Hindu scriptures will also give us a fair idea as to why Darwinian theories were opposed by the Church, and why it may not have created ripples in India. This has nothing to do with India being in the backwaters of science. To repeat myself, however, there is no ground to claim equivalence between

Darwinian evolution and the *Dashavatar*. Describing Kalidasa as the Indian Shakespeare, Caraka's oath as the Indian Hippocratic oath, the *Dashavatar* as the Indian Darwinian theory are all sad examples of imposing Western notions on the Indian psyche.

The fact is, it is bodies and not souls which eventually die a natural death. We cannot do anything about it. Ideas about the self and the person will persist. The body is precious because it creates the circumstances for consciousness to manifest. Even if we accept that consciousness is a product of the biological process, that is, the brain, the body becomes the vehicle for its manifestation. Can consciousness manifest without a body? The immortality of consciousness and its continuity after death is, of course, a matter of debate, but not something to be denied or dismissed out of hand. These questions will continue to bedevil the human mind at least in the foreseeable future, and inspire new philosophies and explanations about human life. They are long-standing mysteries that kindle human creativity and philosophical enquiry into the nature of truth. Even the most advanced science cannot prevent a Nobel laureate at least once in a century to think again about immortality and life after death.

As for evolutionary thought in Hindu traditions, how about *akshad vayu* (physical evolution), *vayoragni* (astrophysical evolution), *agnerapah adbhyah prthvi* (chemical evolution), *prithivyah osadhayah* (biological evolution), *osahibhyo annam* (differentiation of life and the food chain), and *annat purushah* (higher life forms and human evolution)? Of course, the ancient hymn did not anticipate the big bang and evolutionary notions of modern science!

Finally, religion, spirituality and science have grown in different ways in the Islamic, Christian and Hindu worlds. This needs to be studied more carefully and we must avoid generalisations.

MRP: Would it be fair to say that different cultures are good at different kinds of science? For instance, Indians are good at Mathematics and IT, while Jewish Americans of European descent have excelled in theoretical science, and the Japanese are good at miniaturisation, and so on.

PMB: These are ideas paraded for public consumption and have no scientific basis. The first Indian to be elected to The Royal Society (Cursetjee) was a marine engineer and naval architect. And that was in 1841!

PRM: Socio-cultural conditioning may influence activities in science to some extent, but it sounds improbable that different cultures are intrinsically good at different types of science.

MRP: Indian science is often accused of being derivative, unable to ask and frame its own questions, but usually good at replicating or proving what others have already designated as desirable to research. Do you think that a colonial mentality hamstrings our efforts?

PMB: The first statement you made is unfortunately generally true, with notable exceptions. However, this is not on account of a colonial mentality.

PRM: On the face of it, the fact is that India produced some outstanding scientists, like J. C. Bose and C. V. Raman, during the colonial period. Nowadays, an Indian has to become an NRI first to do significant research, let alone win a Nobel Prize!

MRP: Science is supposed to be the pursuit of truth, but in reality we often see it as a handmaiden of a military–industrial–commercial complex, with the state and large corporations calling the shots, deciding what is worth investigating, and where the money should go. Taking our cue from Mahatma Gandhi, to what extent do you think modern science is asuric, that is, controlled and motivated by negative forces?

PMB: Unfortunately, we often confuse science with technology. There are vital differences between the two, which I have enumerated elsewhere. For example, science is the pursuit of truth, but technology is the pursuit, amongst other things, of comfort, convenience, power, and money, which can be for good or for bad.

Science can be bad or mediocre (when done by incompetent scientists), but it can never be 'asuric'. However, technology can be for good or it can be asuric. Numerous examples can be given for both. The decision as to how much money will go into developing asuric technologies is made by a collusion of political and commercial interests.

In practice today, around the world, there is often a nexus between multinational corporations, politicians, bureaucrats, and the rich, directing resources for developing asuric technologies, which benefit a few but harm many, directly or indirectly.

PRM: I would like to add that the practice of confusing spirituality with religion is just as rife and as unfortunate as confusing science and technology. Just as the core of science has to be separated from the envelope of power, politics and commercial exploitation, the core of religion and spirituality has to be extracted from the moss that has accumulated over the years. It is a type of prejudice to think that the evils propagated in the name of science should be excused on account of the political and commercial nexus, but that religion or spirituality are inherently misleading and useless. Religion is the technology of spirituality that proclaims the fundamental unity of existence. Just as technology can be good or bad, religions tend to be good or bad, depending on how grounded they are in the inner spiritual core that forms their basis. The very word 'religion' means to reunite. That religion has more often led to a division in human society is as paradoxical as the fact that science has often led to activities that destroy and exploit humanity.

MRP: How can ethics be wedded to modern scientific pursuits, or are the two separate? Science is considered value-free. Do you agree?

PMB: Scientific truths are indeed value-free. However, the process of doing science generates a whole set of highly desirable values, from honesty and integrity to objectivity, lack of bias and ethics, and many more.

PRM: Indeed! The core of spiritual values enshrined in Indian traditions has also evolved in a similar fashion — as an outcome of the quest for truth.

MRP: Yes, when it comes to India, and perhaps some other societies too, we discover on close examination that both science and spirituality emerge and progress only from this shared quest for truth. At least in that respect they are siblings, even if they occasionally display rivalry, and not aliens or enemies, as it is sometimes thought.

Thank you for sharing your valuable insights.

Note

*This dialogue between an eminent biologist and an Ayurvedic researcher and practitioner exemplifies the difficulties in trying to reconcile modern scientific thinking with any traditional or spiritual approach to healing. The fundamental problem is one of definitions. Dr Bhargava refuses to recognise or accept anything that is 'supernatural'; Dr Ram Manohar, on the other hand, does not believe that the truth about human beings can be entirely contained in the 'physical'. To the latter, 'spirituality' implies the 'trans-physical', something that is beyond, but also permeating in, the physical. To Dr Bhargava, this is an impossibility because everything can be understood in terms of physical nature and its properties. If there is anything 'beyond', then it will one day be understood by instruments similar to those we use to understand the physical. For Dr Ram Manohar, such an approach is reductive, if not dogmatic. If 'spiritual' refers to the soul or spirit, then Dr Bhargava denies its existence. Dr Ram Manohar, instead, uses the word 'consciousness', which modern science also accepts, but usually as a function of the physical organ, the brain. At least when it comes to healing, a patient's attitudes, beliefs, values, and experiences are known to play an important role; these, however, are not easily reducible to any physical or bodily organs of the person. An integrative approach to healing will treat not only the body, but also try to include the 'mind' of the patient. Even if such inclusions are not curative, they have been known to be palliative, especially in terminally ill patients. Science may not accept the existence of a soul or God, but if a patient feels better for believing in such entities, then science would not dismiss such a fact either. Ultimately, this discussion illustrates the different ways in which science may regard certain ideas or beliefs which are as yet 'non-scientific' — either through outright rejection and hostility, tolerant scepticism, or sympathetic understanding.

References

Bhargava, Pushpa M. and Chandana Chakrabarti. 2007. *Angels, Devil, and Science: A Collection of Articles on Scientific Temper*. New Delhi: National Book Trust.

———. 2003. *The Saga of Indian Science since Independence: In a Nutshell*. Hyderabad: Universities Press.

One

Science, Spirituality and Healing

In Search of Definitions

P. Ram Manohar

In Search of Definitions

How do we define these three terms — science, spirituality and healing? In spite of intense discussions and deliberations, it is not clear whether there is a consensus amongst experts on the exact meaning and implications of these terms.

Science has been relatively better defined than spirituality. We can find textbook and working definitions of science that have a clarity not seen in the case of spirituality. More often than not, these terms are used very casually. The expression 'science of spirituality' is most intriguing and complicates things even more. We end up asking questions — can spirituality be a science, can astrology be a science? Or can it be that spirituality and astrology represent approaches that are outside the purview of science?

Additionally, we are also familiar with expressions like 'spiritual science'. This turns the table around and at this stage, we had better find clear definitions if we are to nurture a meaningful dialogue between science and spirituality. There is a need for thoughtful discussions to formally define science and spirituality, so that we do not make the mistake of engaging in serious dialogue with loosely defined concepts.

Epistemological and Ontological Premises of Knowledge Systems

If we look closely into the problem, we can discern that the differences lie in ontological and epistemological premises. At the ontological level, science restricts itself to the physical world, whereas spirituality is the quest to understand the trans-physical realm of existence. Epistemologically, science works with the sense organs and the ordinary wakeful state of the mind as tools to build knowledge. Spirituality, however, claims to invoke higher cognitive faculties of the mind that transcend the jurisdiction of the sense organs.

We encounter a different problem altogether when we try to define and distinguish between science and spirituality in the Indian tradition. It is very difficult to see a clear demarcation between science and spirituality, for example, in the tradition of Ayurveda. Ayurveda is a good example to consider for illustration of this point, because it is a branch of learning in the Indian tradition that displays attributes of science, even as it is not divorced from spiritual moorings. The worldviews of knowledge systems like Ayurveda accommodate science and spirituality within the framework of a continuum that includes the physical and the trans-physical. It seems that the division between science and spirituality has its roots in the Western tradition. As we try to look at it from an Indian perspective, the boundaries disappear and an altogether different approach to knowledge-building emerges on our mindscape.

In the Indian tradition, we encounter what can be described as a knowledge-seeking process. We see that a pluralistic approach to knowledge-building was prevalent in ancient India, and what we understand as science and spirituality would both be accepted as valid approaches to knowledge-building. What we have here is the concept of a knowledge system or *darsana*,[1] which accommodates the approaches of both science and spirituality without really making a watertight distinction between the two.

Carvaka thought and modern science

The closest parallel to science is the knowledge system of Carvaka,[2] which epistemologically restricts the scope of knowledge to the realm of the external senses and the mind, and ontologically restricts reality to the physical world. Carvakas did not believe in the existence of the self after death:

> While life is yours, live joyously;
> None can escape Death's searching eye:
> When once this frame of ours they burn,
> How shall it e'er again return? (Madhava Acharya 1882)[3]

They found no meaning in religious rituals and were categorical in denouncing them:

> If a beast slain in the Jyotishṭoma rite will itself go to heaven,
> Why then does not the sacrificer forthwith offer his own father?

> If the Śráddha produces gratification to beings who are dead,
> Then here, too, in the case of travellers when they start, it is needless to give provisions for the journey.
> If beings in heaven are gratified by our offering the Śráddha here,
> Then why not give food down below to those who are standing on the house-top? (Madhava Acharya 1182)[4]

Carvakas relied upon direct perception as the only valid approach to knowledge, and believed that the goal of life was to live joyfully.

They were also strong antagonists of the caste system and minced no words when it came to voicing their dissent: 'What is this senseless humbug about the castes and the high and low among them when the organs like the mouth, etc in the human body are the same?' (Nambiar 1971: 2.18).

The Carvakas also rejected the notion of the self as separate from the body. According to them, the self is destroyed along with the body. Consciousness is but the by-product of the reactions that take place in the body.[5]

For this reason, this school of thought came to be known as Nastika Darsana. The term Nastika means denial of the other world, the world after death. Carvakas also contended that it is possible to rise to high levels of ethical and moral refinement without the need for religious beliefs and rituals.

On the other hand, the schools of thought that accept the existence of life after death, the immutability of the self when the body is destroyed, came to be known as Astika Darsanas. The term Astika means acceptance of the other world, the *paraloka*.[6] This is exactly the boundary that divides science and spirituality. Paraloka is the transphysical dimension of the human persona as well as the universe.

It needs to be clarified that the allusion to the parallel between modern science and Carvakas is being made with respect to the epistemological and ontological premises, and not with respect to the specific discoveries and inventions that have characterised the development of modern science. It is also not intended to claim that all scientific discoveries and advancements were anticipated in India. Just before the Renaissance in Europe, India was one of the most advanced civilisations in the world in terms of both wealth and scientific advancement (Dharampal 1971). But the development in science that we witnessed in Europe in modern times is without parallel in the known history of humankind.

The Evolution of a Comprehensive Knowledge System in India

The Astika and Nastika schools of thought served as templates that helped to synthesise approaches to understanding the reality that we today refer to as science and spirituality. The confrontations, tensions, exchanges, and interactions between these schools of thought in the cultural history of India set the stage for the development of a worldview that exhibited preparedness for scientific development, and an aspiration for spiritual fulfilment.

It is beyond the scope of this chapter to deliberate on the details of these dialectical oppositions. For the purpose of our discussion, it would suffice to conclude that in India, an intellectual environment prevailed that was conducive to the coexistence of the Nastika and Astika schools, and so in principle, science and spirituality could coexist as valid worldviews. It is important to realise at this juncture that the Astika school became the established worldview, the orthodoxy, and this was crucial in achieving a synthesis. The Astika school of thought was inclusive; it accepted the physical worldview of the Nastika school, but held that there was a reality beyond the physical. The Nastika worldview, on the other hand, was exclusive; it denied outright the existence of the trans-physical. The dominance of the Astika school meant that the Nastika school could also be accepted to a certain extent.[7]

In the course of his commentaries on the Upanishads, Adi Sankaracharya eloquently resolves this conflict through pithy statements: 'Facts of perception cannot be challenged on the ground of improbability because they have been perceived. Perception cannot be nullified by inference and an inference is no authority against perception' (Atmananda 1960: 42).[8] He goes on to say:

> [E]ven the Veda cannot be an authority as against observed facts. Even if hundreds of Vedic texts declare that fire is cold and devoid of light, they cannot become an authority on this point. The Sruti or Veda is merely informative; the scriptures do not intend to alter the nature of things, but to inform about what is unknown as they are. The Veda is an authority in realms of experience that transcend the scope of senses. Here the senses or reason cannot contradict what the Veda informs because it deals with a different sphere of human experience (ibid).[9]

This is the perspective that facilitates the development of a spirituality that can accommodate science, or rather, a spirituality that does not conflict with or oppose science. We do find in the Indian tradition the coexistence of spiritual aspirations and a yearning for scientific advancement.

The *Rig Veda*, for instance, narrates the story of Queen Visphala, who having lost her limbs in a war gets them replaced with artificial limbs and returns to the battlefield (Rigveda 1.116.15).[10] Vedic literature is replete with narrations that resemble science fiction, including stories of organ transplants and other such surgical feats.[11] Puranic lore also contains accounts of technological births that resemble the creation of test-tube babies, cloning, and the like.[12] These are closer to science fiction than myths, even if we admit that such technologies had not been discovered in those days.

It would be an independent exercise altogether to speculate and investigate why science did not develop in India the way it did in Europe.[13] But we cannot forget that some of the breakthroughs that laid the foundation for the development of modern science happened in India in the distant past.[14]

Science and spirituality were both, therefore, pursuits of knowledge, and had little to do in principle with the propagation of dogma. Each was an authority in its own domain and could not pass judgement on the other. It is necessary to point out once again that the distinction between science and spirituality, as we understand them today, did not exist. There were schools of thought that could be compared with science and spirituality. As indicated earlier, the Nastika school of thought represents the template for science and the Astika school of thought, the template for spirituality. It was the Astika school that gained the upper hand and became the orthodoxy, but did not deny the Nastika position — it sought to go beyond it. The emergence of the Astika school created the ground for the synthesis of science and spirituality in India at an early stage, and there was no room for science to develop independently. Ultimately, what prevailed dominantly was what can be characterised as a knowledge system, one that was spiritually oriented when dealing with science and scientifically oriented when dealing with spirituality. Perhaps this is the reason why science did not develop in India the way it did in the West, but it did create an atmosphere that was always ready for science, an intellectual inclination that aspired for science.

Adi Sankara's remarks are quite revealing in this context. He says:

> The test of the authority or otherwise of a passage is not whether it states a fact or an action, but its capacity to generate indubitable and fruitful knowledge. A passage that has this is authoritative and one that lacks it is not (Atmananda 1960: 35).[15]

He makes a clear distinction between speculation and objective knowledge based on experience: 'Perception of the true nature of reality is not a product of man's intellect. It depends on the nature of the object' (ibid.).

He then goes on to demarcate the domain of spirituality: 'The Yogis can perceive with the mind alone, without the aid of senses'; and 'In its own sphere, Vedas have independent authority and need no other support just as the Sun in the sphere of forms' (ibid.).[16]

Be it the domain of the physical world or the trans-physical, there was no place for mere speculation or imagination. The fact that the Astika school of thought dominated in India led to the emergence of a knowledge system that was predominantly spiritual in outlook, although this was supplemented with a scientific approach to understanding the mundane world. Amongst the Nastika schools, Buddhism and Jainism were well-codified and developed into organised establishments. It is pertinent to note that the Carvaka school or Lokayata, as it was also known, never became established as a predominant school of thought. In fact, there are no primary sources on Carvaka Darasana available today. But the Carvaka system of thought exerted a powerful influence and helped to achieve a balance between the spiritual and material worldviews. The Carvaka school ensured that the materialistic perspective also found a legitimate place in the canvas depicting reality. In the tradition of Ayurveda, we can see the implications of this influence. The *Caraka Samhita* proclaims that one must protect one's body at all costs and that everything is lost when the body is destroyed.[17] The *Sushruta Samhita* says that in therapeutics, one does not think beyond the realm of the five elements.[18] We find epistemology and ontology reaching out to the trans-physical realm of existence, and being less fixed on the physical. Yet there was no conflict between the two, and no exclusivist attitude.

Ayurveda as an Example of a Complete Knowledge System

Ayurveda is a rather unique example of a knowledge system that developed in the Indian cultural milieu, and gave more or less equal attention to both the physical and trans-physical dimensions of reality.[19] In fact, Ayurveda has a more pronounced focus on the physical dimension of reality, even as it embraces trans-physical aspects of life to understand health and disease in a comprehensive manner.[20]

We can thus construct a model of reality inspired by the tradition of Ayurveda, which will work as an interface between science and spirituality, something that we can refer to as a knowledge system without dividing it into science and spirituality.

Ayurveda has constructed a three-dimensional view of reality comprising of the physical (*adhibhautika*), mental (*adhidaivika*), and transcendental (*adhyatma*) realms of existence.[21] At the level of the microcosm, they correspond to the body (*sarira*), mind (*satva*) and self (*atma*).[22] Sub-divisions are possible within this scheme, but they can ultimately be resolved into the trinity of the body, mind and self. For example, the three-dimensional view of the human being can be expanded into the five sheaths of the Upanishads. The Food Sheath corresponds to the physical body, the Mind Sheath to the Mind itself, and the Bliss Sheath to the Self. The Vital Sheath from an Ayurvedic perspective is the unstable link between the Body and the Mind, and is simply called *prana*. The mind connects to the body through *prana*. Life exists as long as *prana* maintains the connection between the body and the mind. Death happens when this link is broken and the physical body disintegrates. The Sheath of Intelligence is simply called *buddhi* in Ayurveda. This is the link between the mind and the self, which causes individuation. When the link between the mind and the self is dissolved, the individual self dissolves and is liberated — *moksa*.[23] The goal of Ayurveda is to preserve and prolong the connection between the Body and the Mind (*Laukiki Cikitsa*), and work for the dissolution of the Mind in the Self before death catches up eventually (*Naisthiki Cikitsa*).[24]

From an epistemological point of view, these three realms of reality are tangible (*vyakta*), partially tangible (*vyaktavyakta*), and intangible (*avyakta*).[25] The tangible realm of the physical world can be experienced and understood by direct perception (*pratyaksa*). The partially tangible realm of the physical as well as mental worlds can be experienced and understood by inference (*anumana*). The intangible realm can be experienced and understood only by invoking heightened states of awareness (*alaukikapratyaksa*), or through the words of individuals who have succeeded in doing so.[26]

There are three types of treatment in Ayurveda — that which operates at the physical level and is empirico-rational, known as Yuktivyapasraya; that which operates at the mental level and aims to invoke the innate self-healing powers of the individual, known as Satvavajaya; and finally, that which operates from outside and relies on healing powers beyond the scope of rational medical interventions, known as Daivavyapasraya.[27]

Ayurveda is truly the most ancient model of integrative medicine that seeks to harmonise body, mind and self, both from within and without, at the physical, mental and transcendental realms of existence.

The three-dimensional epistemological and ontological premises on which Ayurveda has been erected as a knowledge system can help us to sketch a panoramic view of reality, in which science and spirituality coalesce into one complete knowledge system. Table 1.1 illustrates this model with a few examples.

Table 1.1: Three-dimensional view of human aspirations

Intangible	*Partially Tangible*	*Tangible*
Transcendental	Mental	Physical
Self	Mind	Body
Causal	Subtle	Gross
Cittam	Satva Rajas Tamas	Vata Pitta Kapha
Adhyatmika	Adhidaivika	Adhibhautika
Yoga	Jyotisha	Ayurveda
Religion, Spirituality, Parapsychology	Psychology, Sociology, Anthropology	Physical Science, Biology, Medicine
Wellness	Health	Life
Trans Science	Soft Science	Hard Science

What we have here is a system of correspondence that correlates epistemological and ontological entities on the canvas of a three-dimensional view of existence. There is a space for all human aspirations, ranging from hard-core science to the most intense experience of spirituality.

Scientific Rigour in Ayurveda

Ayurveda has emphasised the need for adopting a fundamentally scientific and rational approach to healing, which it terms *yuktivya-pashraya*. However, this approach can be supplemented with other modalities and approaches. Thus, according to Ayurveda, prayer can be an adjuvant therapy to a typical medical intervention. But prayer is never the frontline or stand-alone approach to treatment.

Classical Ayurvedic texts emphasise that clinical outcomes should be substantiated with proper evidence and reasoning. The chance effect of a medicine should be ruled out by rigorous analysis of the cause and effect relationship.[28]

Ayurveda is perhaps the first medical system in the world to point out that many diseases are self-limiting, that is, they resolve without any treatment. Ayurveda also mentions that the mind can be influenced to promote healing (placebo), and it also talks about spontaneous remission. The physician is cautioned against making false claims of success by treating such conditions.

Clinical evidence is built on the basis of observations (*anumana*) and experimentation (*yukti*).[29] A cause and effect relationship is established by going beyond coincidence (*sahacharya*) and correlation (*vyapti*) to causation (*hetu*). Causation is established through tests of significance, like Specificity (*avyabhicaritva*) and Sensitivity (*avinabhavasambandha*). When a causal relationship is suspected (*paksa*), it should be compared with a positive control (*sapaksa*) and negative control (*vipaksa*), which is very similar to the design of a clinical trial in modern research.

It is beyond the scope of this chapter to examine in detail the scientific rigour in the tradition of Ayurveda. Ayurveda preserved its stature as a rational system of healing, even as it embraced spiritual dimensions of health and wellbeing.

The Definition of Healing and Rediscovery of a Complete Knowledge System

We have to now look at the definition of healing. What is healing? Healing is restoration of wholeness; integrating the parts to make it a composite whole again. It is a process that is initiated from the depths of one's being, and results in a psycho-spiritual transformation of the individual. It is not mere elimination of physical disease. It is the integration of body, mind and self to sustain life, establish health, and nurture wellness.[30] Healing has no meaning in a worldview engrossed only with the physical aspects of the human being or the universe.

The need to recognise the three dimensions of the human persona is being felt more in the field of medicine than in any other discipline. Even if it is not fully mainstream yet, integrative medicine has become the watchword to discover a more complete form of health care. And integrative medicine means harmonising the body, mind and self.[31]

It appears as though the seeds for a future synthesis of science and spirituality are being sown in the field of medicine and health care. The complexities of the human personality and its implications in health and disease are forcing a re-examination of the reductionist approach of modern science, which has underpinned the development of bio-medicine. One of the oldest medical systems in the world remains a living example and proof that such an approach is viable, and can bring a human touch to health care and a transformation of personality that can help us to discover better and more wholesome ways to achieve health and wellness.

The science and spirituality of healing might well become the platform for the creation of a comprehensive approach to knowledge and liberation in contemporary times.

Notes

1. The word *darsana* in Sanskrit means 'to see'. It is derived from the root *dṛś*, 'to see'. In the context of knowledge, it denotes the worldviews embodied in different schools of Indian thought.
2. *Carvaka* means 'pleasing speech' (*caru ramaniyo vaka uktiryasya sa carvakah*) and denotes the materialistic and atheistic school of thought prevalent in ancient India. According to historians, it may have originated in the *Barhaspatya Sutras* of Brihaspati. The school is named after Carvaka, who was supposedly a disciple of Brihaspati. This school of thought was also known as *Lokayata* (*loka ayatam prasrtamityarthah*), which means the prevalent worldview of the common people.
3. This famous Carvaka teaching beckons humankind to live a life of luxury and pleasure, even at the cost of running into debt — *yavajjivet sukham jivet rnam krtva ghrtam pibet, bhasmibhutasya dehasya punaragamanam kutah*. This, and all further quotations from the *Sarva-Darsana-Samgraha*, are excerpted from the Project Gutenberg ebook of Madhava Acharya's original, translated by E. B. Cowell and A. E. Gough (http://www.gutenberg.org/files/34125/34125-h/34125-h.htm; accessed 8 September 2011).

4. These verses vehemently attack the practice of animal slaughter for religious purposes, as well as the system of offering food to the deceased — *pasuscennihatah svargam jyotistome gamisyati, svapita yajamanena tatra kasmanna himsyate; svargasthita yada trptim gaccheyustatra danatah, prasadasyoparisthanamatra kasmanna diyate.*
5. The Carvaka school categorically dismisses the idea of an individual soul by stating that consciousness is but a by-product of material processes, an epiphenomenon of matter — *tatraprthivyadinibhutanicatvaritattvani. Tebhyaevadehakaraparinatebhyahkinvadibhyomadsaktivaccaitanyamupajayate.*
6. The Nastika schools deny the existence of the trans-physical world expounded in the Vedas, while the Astika schools accept this viewpoint — *nasti vedodito loka iti yesam matih sthira, nastikaste tathastiti matiryesam ta astikah.*
7. Sayana argues in the *Sarvadarshansamgraha* that it is difficult to reject Carvaka Darsana because its arguments are powerful — *durucchedam hi carvakasyacestitam.*
8. In his commentary on the *Bhagavad Gita* (pp. 18–66), Sankara denies the authority of the Vedas to pass judgement in matters of the physical world. If the Vedas make a statement that is contradicted by actual observations, then that statement has to be rejected as invalid — *na ca pratyaksavirodhe sruteh pramanyam, na hi srutisatamapi sitogniraprakasa iti bruvat pramanyam labhate.*
9. In his commentary on the *Brihadaranyaka Upanisad*, Sankara clarifies that the scriptures attempt to reveal the nature of objects as they are. The function of the scripture is to reveal what is unknown and not to distort reality — *sruteh jnapakatvat, na sastram padarthan anyathakartum pravrttam kim tarhi yathabhutanamajnatanam jnapane.*
10. The *Rig Veda* describes the encounter of Queen Visphala in a battle and the replacement of her severed legs with iron limbs — *caritram hi verivachediparnamajakhelasyaparitakmyayam, sadyojanghamayasam vispalayaidhanehitesartavepratyadhattam.*
11. The *Caraka Samhita*, a celebrated text of Ayurveda, recounts the Vedic narratives of organ transplantation, artificial dentures and eye transplant — *asvinau devabhisajau yajnavahaviti smrtau yajnasya hi siraschinnam punastabhyam samahitam, prasirna dasanah pusno netre naste bhagasya ca, vajrinasca bhujastambhastabhyameva cikitsitah.*
12. Stories about what can be termed technological births abound in Puranic lore. The Kauravas were born by splitting a lump of flesh delivered by Gandhari into 101 pieces; Kartikeya developed outside the womb of Parvati; Sage Agastya was born from a pot. All these stories refer to the possibility of extra-uterine fertilisation, extra-uterine gestation, cloning, and other such technology-assisted births. These can perhaps be considered the earliest science fiction accounts in the Indian tradition.

13. Many modern scholars have contended that the dominance of religion led to the decline of science in India, just like in the West (see Chattopadhyaya 1977). It is, however, pertinent to note that on the eve of colonialism, science and technology in India was much more advanced than in Europe. There is room to speculate that the failure of the Indian civilisational process to modernise itself like Europe during the Renaissance period led to the stagnation of science in modern India.
14. See Basham (2004), and Majumdar and Pusalker (1951). These landmark publications replaced imperialist views on Indian history, and highlighted the great contributions made by Indian civilisation towards the progress of science.
15. In the course of his commentary on the *Brhadaranyakopanisad*, Sankara defines what can be termed the ultimate objective criterion for deciding the validity or otherwise of a statement: it should be able to generate knowledge that can be meaningfully applied in practice — *na hi vakyasya vastvanvyakhyam kriyanvakhyanam va pramanyapramanyakaranam. kim tarhi, niscitaphalavadvijnanotpadakatvam. tadyatrasti tadpramanam vakyam, yatra nasti tadapramanam.*
16. Sankara clarifies that practitioners of yoga can perceive directly through the mind without the aid of sense organs, and that Vedic scriptures constitute the source for knowledge that transcends the realm of the senses — *mana eva kevalam rupajnananimittam yoginam, srutisca nah pramanam atindriyavisayavijnanotpattau.*
17. The *Caraka Samhita* issues a categorical warning underlining the need to protect one's body at all costs. When the body is gone, everything is lost — *sarvamanyatparityajyasariramanupalayet, tadabhave hi bhavanam sarvabhavahsaririnam.*
18. Susruta, the pioneering surgeon in the tradition of Ayurveda, points out that in the context of treatment, one does not have to think beyond the five elements — *bhutebhyo hi paramyasmatnasticintacikitsite.*
19. There is a very interesting debate in the *Caraka Samhita* on the plausibility of the notion of a trans-physical realm of existence. The text attempts to rationalise the concept of trans-physical reality by providing evidence in the form of direct perception, perception-aided inference, testimonials of authorities, and experimentation.
20. Ayurveda makes it clear that its focus is restricted to the embodied individual. Although it accepts the trans-physical dimensions of the human personality, it works on the physical realm — *sa puman cetanam tacca taccadhikaranam matam, vedasyasya yadarthohi vedoyam samprakasitah.*
21. Susruta elaborates the three-dimensional nature of reality by referring to the *adhibhautika, adhyatmika* and *adhidaivika* realms of existence — *svah svascaisam visayo adhibhutam svayamadhyatmam, adhidaivatam.*
22. The body, mind and self are considered the tripod on which the life process manifests and sustains itself — *sattvamatma sariram ca trayametat tridandavat, lokastishtati samyogat tatra sarvam pratishtitam.*

23. When the individual self dissolves, only the consciousness of Brahman remains. There is no scope for individuated existence — *atah param brahmabhuto bhutatma nopalabhyate, nihsrtah sarvabhavebhyascihnam yasya na vidyate.*
24. The treatment that helps to dissolve the mind in the self is the permanent cure for all illnesses — *cikitsa tu naistiki ya vinopadham.*
25. Reality is mapped as the subject and object which expands into the tangible, intangible, and partially tangible realms of existence — *iti ksetram samuddistam sarvamavyaktavarjitam, avyaktamasya ksetrasya ksetrajnamrsayo viduh.*
26. The sages of yore discovered the deeper knowledge of Ayurveda through the inner eye of knowledge in a state of meditation — *maharsayaste dadrsuh yathavajjnanacaksusa.*
27. Treatment is of three kinds, depending on whether it harnesses the physical, mental, or spiritual energies: *trividhamausadhamiti — daivavyapasrayam, yuktivyapasrayam, sattvavajayasceti.*
28. The *Caraka Samhita* minces no words to emphasise the need for a rational and evidence-based approach to clinical practice when it says that clinical events have specific causes, and that clinical treatment outcomes should be substantiated with proper observations and reasoning to rule out the chance effect of medications — *vina tarkena ya siddhiryadrcchasiddhireva sa, sarvam tadhetuvasagam hetorabhavannanuvartate.*
29. The process of *yukti* aims to understand the multiple factors working behind a given phenomenon, the manipulation of which can bring the event under one's control — *buddhih pasyati ya bhavan bahukaranayogajan, yuktistrikala sa jneya.*
30. The classical Ayurvedic texts provide the earliest concepts of integrative medicine. In the *Susruta Samhita*, the healthy individual is defined as one who is established in the self integrated harmoniously with the mind, sense organs and the body — *samadosah samagnisca samadhatumalakriyah, prasannatmendriyamanah svastha ityabhidhiyate.*
31. 'Integrative medicine' is a term that denotes the combination of the practices and methods of alternative medicine with conventional medicine. Since such approaches lay emphasis on body and mind, integrative medicine has also come to be known as the approach that integrates body, mind and spirit.

References

Atmananda, Swami. 1960. *Sankara's Teachings in His Own Words*. Mumbai: Bharatiya Vidya Bhavan.

Basham, Arthur Llewellyn. 2004. *The Wonder that Was India*. London: Picador.

Chattopadhyaya, Debiprasad. 1977. *Science and Society in Ancient India*. Kolkata: Research India Publications.

Dharampal. 1971. *Indian Science and Technology in the Eighteenth Century: Some Contemporary European Accounts*. New Delhi: Impex India.

Madhava Acharya. 1882. *The Sarva-Darsana-Samgraha or Review of the Different Systems of Hindu Philosophy* (E. B. Cowell and A. E. Gough, trans.). London: Trübner and Co. (Project Gutenberg eBook).

Majumdar, R. C. and A. D. Pusalker. 1951. *The History and Culture of the Indian People*. Bombay [Mumbai]: Bharatiya Vidya Bhavan.

Nambiar, Sita Krishna. 1971. *Prabodhacandrodaya of Krsna Misra*. New Delhi: Motilal Banarasidass.

Tripati, Acharya Kedaranatha. 1985. *tarkasaMgraha: nyAyabodhinI Sanskrit and Hindi vyAkhyAna*. Varanasi: Kashi Hindu Viswavidyalaya.

Yadavji Trikamji Acharya (ed.). 2002. *Caraka Samhita*. Varanasi: Chaukhambha Surabharati.

———. 1994. *Sushruta Samhita*. Varanasi: Chaukhambha Surabharati.

Two

Beyond Mind–Body Medicine

Ramesh Bijlani

The 20th century was an extremely eventful period in the history of modern medicine. The first half of the century was marked by spectacular advances such as the conquest of infectious diseases and nutritional deficiencies, the discovery of insulin and X-rays, and the advent of safe and painless surgery. As a result, the countries that benefitted the most from these advances experienced a doubling of life expectancy. But the availability of powerful new tools also pushed the mind–body relationship into oblivion. Antibiotics, vitamins, or insulin do not depend for their efficacy on what is going on in the patient's mind. However, the euphoria generated by these remarkable achievements did not last long. Infectious diseases and vitamin deficiencies, which used to kill people young, were replaced with heart disease and cancer, which affect people of all ages. Further, the new killers of humankind did not lend themselves to a mechanistic approach the way the old killers had. It was discovered that the roots of the new killers lay in the modern lifestyle, of which mental stress is a major accompaniment. Studies that approached the issue from a variety of angles all led to the general conclusion that mental stress makes an overriding contribution to lifestyle disorders. Epidemiological studies were done on university students who were given questionnaires to assess their stress levels, and follow-up studies were conducted 30–35 years later. These studies revealed that only about half of those who were mentally well-adjusted in their youth contracted mid-life illnesses such as high blood pressure, heart disease, duodenal ulcer, and alcoholism. On the other hand, almost every single person who was mentally maladjusted in youth was found to have at least one mid-life disease 30–35 years later (Russek and Schwartz 1997: 144–49).

Rabbits placed on a high-cholesterol diet could be protected from the harmful effects of the diet by a daily dose of petting and being played with (Nerem et al. 1980: 1475–76). Examination stress or bereavement was found to depress immunocompetence (Kiecolt-Glaser et al. 2002: 83–107). If mental stress could cause illness, could love, hope and laughter lead to recovery, was the simple question asked — not by a doctor, but a wise patient, Norman Cousins. Norman Cousins became his own guinea pig, and recovered from an essentially incurable disease, ankylosing spondylitis, by using a combination of laughter and vitamin C (Cousins 1979). This paved the way for a large number of scientific studies and the emergence of a new discipline called Psychoneuroimmunology. Lifestyle modification and mental relaxation based on Yoga were found to help those with coronary heart disease (Gould et al. 1995: 894–901), and a weekly psychosocial intervention improved the survival of women with stage IV metastatic breast cancer (Spiegel et al. 1989: 888–91). The overall result of these wide-ranging studies was the emergence of a new era in modern medicine during the second half of the 20th century — the era of mind–body medicine (Dossey 1993).

Mind-Body Medicine

Without rejecting the achievements of physical medicine, mind–body medicine has added a new dimension to modern medicine. Mind–body medicine recognises the remarkable extent to which the patient can use the powers of his own mind to heal his body. It is now well known that the body has a tremendous capacity for self-healing (Brownstein 2005). However, to make the best use of this capacity, optimum conditions have to be created for the self-healing mechanisms to work. These conditions are, in general, the opposite of those which led to the disease in the first place. In the case of lifestyle disorders, self-healing is therefore promoted by a healthy lifestyle and mental peace. Further, self-healing is facilitated if the patient believes in the ability of the body to heal itself, and has faith in the physician and the treatment. Given these conditions, a healer can awaken the patient to the tremendous capacity of the body to repair itself, and help the patient use his own inner resources to recover from an illness. Nearly 100 years ago, Sri Aurobindo wrote: 'It should take long for self-cure to replace medicine, because of the fear, self-distrust and unnatural physical reliance on drugs which medical science has taught to our minds and bodies and made our second nature' (The Mother 2001 [1977] : 325). Mind–body medicine has fulfilled Sri Aurobindo's vision by reducing our excessive dependence on drugs and other external interventions. Instead, mind–body medicine relies considerably on the pharmacy residing in the body itself, which is the best pharmacy by far (Chopra 1989).

Mind–Body Medicine and the Spiritual Worldview

The scientific discoveries pointing to an intimate connection between the body and the mind, which have created a new wave in modern medicine, are in fact natural corollaries of the spiritual worldview. In essence, a spiritual worldview considers all creation the manifestation of the One Infinite Creator, and believes that the Spirit of the Creator pervades all creation. From this view, it follows that different parts of the being, such as the body, mind and intellect, are different modes of expression of the same Supreme Consciousness. Hence, the effect of the mind on the body, or vice versa, represents merely the effect of one mode of Consciousness on another. Similarly, using the powers of the mind to heal the body — be it through faith in the physician, belief in self-healing, or through imagery — also amounts to using one mode of Consciousness to correct a disorder in another mode of Consciousness (Chopra 1989).

Beyond Mind–Body Medicine

The implications of this spiritual worldview, when applied to healing, go far beyond mind–body medicine. The body and mind of an individual are just two modes of expression of that Supreme Consciousness. The bodies and minds of healers and those of the other well-wishers of the patient are also manifestations of the same Supreme Consciousness. Further, the Supreme Consciousness resides in all creation — animate and inanimate — in the form of the invisible but universal all-pervasive spirit. Thus, the spirit of the individual (the soul) is connected with the spirit of the air (and the subtle body) surrounding the individual, which in turn is continuous with the souls of the other individuals. Hence, the boundary of the individual defined by the skin is only a partial reality. What connects the individual with everything and everyone around him is the spirit, which is unique in being neither matter nor energy, neither particulate nor a waveform. However, the spirit provides a continuity which allows immediate, unmediated and unmitigated communication. For want of a better science-friendly word, the communication is sometimes said to depend on transmission of 'energy', or to travel through an 'energy field'. A healer can use this mode of communication to lend a helping hand to the self-healing mechanisms of the patient. Just as the mind of the patient can affect his body, the mind of the healer should also be able to affect the body of the patient because of their being interconnected through the Universal Spirit. Using the same channel, the prayers and empathic concern of the patient's well-wishers should be able to help the patient too. Since the influence based on spiritual interconnectedness is immediate and its intensity not affected by distance, the effectiveness of the healing intentions and prayers should be irrespective of physical distance between the healer or well-wishers, and the patient. This is the plausible basis of various therapies such as therapeutic touch, distance healing and intercessory prayer. In therapeutic touch, the healer's hand acts as a visible conduit for his healing intentions. But such a physical connection does not seem to be strictly necessary. In distance healing, the changes initiated by the healing intentions in the 'energy field' that unites the healer with the patient can affect the patient favourably, irrespective of the distance separating the two. Scientific medicine is now open to these possibilities and is ready to look at studies examining these modalities of treatment.

The Evidence So Far

Studies examining the efficacy of intercessory prayer on healing have recently shown an exponential increase (Bijlani 2006: 171–87; Dossey 1999). The most cited studies have used the design of a double-blind randomised controlled trial (Byrd 1988: 826–29; Harris et al. 1999: 2273–78). The results have, in general, been weakly positive. Although a randomised controlled trial is the gold standard for assessing the efficacy of a drug, such a trial is inappropriate for studying the efficacy of prayer. Further, a foolproof experimental design for studying the efficacy of prayer seems to be impossible (Chibnall 2001: 2529–36). Finally, even if prayer works, it always remains doubtful whether prayer itself promotes the biological process of healing. It is impossible to rule out the possibility that the patient gets better because of his faith in the prayer. In that case, the improvement is attributable to the effect of the patient's mind on his own body rather than to somebody else's prayers.

It may be assumed that animals do not believe in prayer or spiritual healing. Hence, animal studies are more suitable than human studies for settling the question of whether the treatment itself is effective, or if it works because the patient believes that it will work. In an interesting study, uniform surgical wounds were created in three groups of mice. The cages of one of these groups were held up for 15 minutes at a time twice a day by a spiritual healer who tried to heal the wounds by mental means. The cages of the second group of mice were not held by the healer, but were maintained at the same temperature as the cages being held. The mice in the third group were neither held by the healer nor received the additional heating. Observations made after 14 days revealed that wounds in the experimental group had healed much faster than in the control groups (Chibnall 2001).

It may, however, be argued that animals also appreciate getting special attention, such as that involved in their cage being held by a gentle soul. Thus, the faster healing may reflect their mind–body relationship working in favour of healing, rather than the spiritual effect of the cage being held by a healer. Therefore, plant studies may be more convincing than animal studies. In a certain experiment, barley seeds were damaged by watering them with a 1 per cent saline solution. In the experimental group, an effort was made to minimise the damaging effect of salinity by a healer holding the beaker containing the solution. The seeds watered with the healer-held saline grew better than those watered with the control saline of the same concentration; the difference was statistically significant (Grad 1965: 195–27).

However, plants do have a rudimentary consciousness, and they may respond to love and attention in ways similar to humans and animals. Therefore, experiments made with tissues, cells and enzyme systems may give us a more definitive insight into the biological effects of willing, wishing, intentionality, and prayer. One study examined the effect of protective intentions based on visualisation on the haemolysis (breakdown) of red blood cells suspended in test tubes containing a hypotonic (weak) salt solution. Although the 'energy' for protection was sent mentally by unskilled persons, the protective effect was statistically significant (Braud 1990: 1–24). A recent study examined the effect of psychosomatic power emitted through Zen meditation on prostate cancer cells. It was found that the experimental treatment significantly reduced the growth rate and enhanced the expression of a differentiation antigen in the cancer cells (Yu et al. 2003: 499–507). Positive results have frequently been reported regarding the healer's ability to influence (positively or negatively) the growth of fungi or bacteria, the rate of mutation of *Escherichia coli*, or the activity of enzyme systems in test tubes. Several such studies have been reviewed by Astin et al. (2000: 903–10), Benor (1990: 9–33), Dossey (1993, 1999), and Miovic (2003: 7–21).

Conclusion

Medicine has finally crossed some sacrosanct self-imposed boundaries. In the scheme of physical medicine — as seen in L. Dossey's Era I medicine (1999) — a drug or a surgical intervention was considered the most essential part of the treatment. Mind–body medicine — Era II medicine (ibid.) — added to the physician's physical armamentarium, the patient's own mental resources. However, scientists continued to interpret the efficacy of mind–body medicine in mechanistic terms. It was explained entirely in terms of the chemicals released by the brain, which in turn could enhance the immunocompetence of the patient, or trigger the release of healing molecules from the patient's endogenous pharmacy. But from the spiritual point of view, the brain is only a mechanism for giving a chemical form to the changes initiated in the consciousness of the person. Further, the consciousness of a person is co-extensive with the consciousness of his fellow beings. Hence, the consciousness of the patient's fellow beings may also be able to initiate a favourable change in the patient's body. This possibility, however irrational and incredible it appears, is consistent with observations made across a broad spectrum covering people, plants and Petri dishes. The crumbling of the barriers restricting our imagination was obvious when the Mecca of modern medicine, Boston, hosted at Harvard, in December 1997, a conference on 'Intercessory Prayer and Distant Healing Intentions: Clinical and Laboratory Research'. About 100 medical scientists participated in the conference and shared their research on a subject which was, till recently, a taboo in modern medicine. Providence-based medicine is rapidly becoming an integral part of evidence-based medicine. Sri Aurobindo's exhortation from nearly 100 years ago bears remembering here: 'Unappalled by the fear of death canst thou leave to Him, not as an experiment, with a calm and entire faith thy ailments? Thou shalt find that in the end He exceeds the skill of a million doctors' (The Mother 2001 [1977]: 324).

References

Astin, J. A., E. Harkness and E. Ernst. 2000. 'The Efficacy of "Distant Healing": A Systematic Review of Randomized Trials', *Annals of Internal Medicine*, 132: 903–10.

Benor, D. J. 1990. 'Survey of Spiritual Healing Research', *Complementary Medical Research*, 4: 9–33.

Bijlani, R. 2006. 'A Critical Look at the Evidence Linking Prayer and Healing', in K. Pandikattu (ed.), *Together Towards Tomorrow: Interfacing Science and Religion in India. Essays in Honour of Professor Job Kozhamthadam S. J.* Pune: Association of Science, Society and Religion.

Braud, W. G. 1990. 'Distant Mental Influence on Rate of Hemolysis of Human Red Blood Cells', *Journal of the American Society for Psychical Research*, 84 (1): 1–24.

Brownstein, A. 2005. *Extraordinary Healing: The Amazing Power of Your Body's Secret Healing System.* Gig Harbor: Harbor Press.

Byrd, R. J. 1988. 'Positive Therapeutic Effects of Intercessory Prayer in a Coronary Care Unit Population', *Southern Medical Journal*, 81: 826–29.

Chibnall, J. T. 2001. 'Experiments on Distant Intercessory Prayer: God, Science and the Lesson of Massah', *Archives of Internal Medicine*, 161: 2529–36.

Chopra, D. 1989. *Quantum Healing: Exploring the Frontiers of Mind/Body Medicine.* New York: Bantam Books.

Cousins, N. 1979. *The Anatomy of an Illness as Perceived by the Patient.* New York: W. W. Norton.

Dossey, L. 1993. *Healing Words: The Power of Prayer and the Practice of Medicine.* New York: Harper Collins.

———. 1999. *Reinventing Medicine: Beyond Mind-Body to a New Era of Healing.* New York: Harper San Fransisco.

Gould, K. L., D. Ornish, L. Scherwitz, S. Brown, R. P. Edens, M. J. Hess, N. Mullani, L. Bolomy, F. Dobbs, W. T. Armstrong, T. Merritt, T. Ports, S. Sparler, and J. Billings. 1995. 'Changes in Myocardial Perfusion Abnormalities by Positron Emission Tomography after Long Term, Intense Risk Factor Modification', *JAMA: The Journal of the American Medical Association*, 274: 894–901.

Grad, B. R. 1965. 'Some Biological Effects of Laying-on of Hands: A Review of Experiments with Animals and Plants', *Journal of the American Society for Psychical Research*, 59: 95–127.

Harris, W. S., M. Gowda, J. W. Kolb, C. P. Strychacz, J. L. Vacek, P. G. Jones, A. Forker, J. H. O'Keefe, and B. D. McCallister. 1999. 'A Randomized, Controlled Trial of the Effects of Remote, Intercessory Prayer on Outcomes in Patients Admitted to the Coronary Care Unit', *Archives of Internal Medicine*, 159: 2273–78.

Kiecolt-Glaser, J. K., L. McGuire, T. F. Robles, and R. Glaser. 2002. 'Emotions, Morbidity, and Mortality: New Perspectives from Psychoneuroimmunology', *Annual Review of Psychology*, 53: 83–107.

Miovic, M. 2003. 'Non-local Studies — Implications for Health', *NAMAH: New Approaches to Medicine and Health*, 11 (1): 7–21.

Mother, The. 2001 [1977]. *On Thoughts and Aphorisms*. Pondicherry (Puducherry): Sri Aurobindo Ashram Publication Department.

Nerem, R. M., M. J. Levesque and J. F. Cornhill. 1980. 'Social Environment as a Factor in Diet-induced Atherosclerosi', *Science*, 208 (4451): 1475–76.

Russek, L. G., and G. E. Schwartz. 1997. 'Perceptions of Parental Caring Predict Health Status in Midlife: A 35-year Follow-up of the Harvard Mastery of Stress Study', *Psychosomatic Medicine*, 59: 144–49.

Spiegel, D., J. R. Bloom, H. C. Kraemer, and E. Gottheil. 1989. 'Effect of Psychosocial Treatment on Survival of Patients with Metastatic Breast Cancer', *Lancet*, 2: 888–91.

Yu, T., H. L. Tsai and M. L. Hwang. 2003. 'Suppressing Tumor Progression of In Vitro Prostate Cancer Cells by Emitted Psychosomatic Power through Zen Meditation', *The American Journal of Chinese Medicine*, 31: 499–507.

Three

Spirituality and Health

O. P. Yadava

Traditionally, and since time immemorial, spirituality has been an integral component of health care. However, the fast-paced technological advances of the past 100 years have changed the focus of health care from a caring, service-oriented, holistic model to a technological, cure-oriented, impersonal one. The past couple of decades have seen a resurgence of attempts oriented towards restoring medicine to its spiritual roots.

Disease and suffering are not just physical phenomena, but multidimensional ones, and often encompass mental, social, spiritual, and existential elements. In most cultures of the world, body and soul have always been viewed as composite and integral components of an individual, and there has been no conception of a dichotomy between the two. In ancient times, both were ministered to by a common individual, like the shaman of North Europe and Siberia, who fulfilled the role of both priest and healer. Closer to our times, Jesus Christ was regarded as a healer of both the body and the spirit. However, due to modern advances, from the 17th century onwards there has been a divergence in the two components of health — spiritual and physical. The philosophy of modern medicine can be attributed to Rene Descartes, a 17th-century philosopher, who believed that the world operated according to mechanical laws, without reference to meaning and purpose (Droege 1991). Thus evolved what we practice today as the bio-medical model of the delivery of medicine, in which physicians are trained to be objective and scientific, and in which the element of spirituality has no role in the diagnostic or therapeutic armamentarium of the physician. Such practices led to the development of the 'science of medicine', but to the peril of the 'art of medicine'. I do not want to decry scientific progress, but today, the art of medicine has equal, if not more, relevance and importance than the science of medicine in the task of providing a compassionate, caring, and healing touch to ailing multitudes all over the world. As Dr Christina Puchalski of George Washington University Medical Center once said, 'Our work as clinicians goes beyond making the correct diagnosis to partnering with our patients to help them through their suffering' (2004).

Here, one needs to differentiate between 'healing' and 'cure'. In modern medicine, disease is viewed as the disruption of the normal physiology, and treatment attempts to restore objective deficits. However, as Puchalski said, 'healing involves more than just technical fixes' (2001b: 32). Although cure looks after the physical component, healing is more encompassing and restores the individual to a state of 'wholeness'. To quote E. J. Cassell, 'In suffering, disruption of the whole person is the dominant theme' (2003: 199). It is here that spirituality plays its greatest role, by healing an individual as a whole, rather than curing just a part of him; indeed, most illnesses do not really have a cure. A person may look to medical care to alleviate his sufferings, but when allopathy fails, he begins to look towards alternate medicine and to spirituality for meaning, purpose and understanding. Viktor Frankl, a psychiatrist during World War II in the Nazi concentration camps, commented, 'Man is not destroyed by suffering, he is destroyed by suffering without meaning' (Puchalski 2001a: 352). He noticed that the prisoners of the concentration camps could cope with their suffering when they found meaning in it, and it is in this respect that spirituality effects a true healing. For example, even in a dying patient, transcendental and meaningful experiences can restore a sense of wholeness by attending to the patient's spiritual needs and beliefs; even though the patient may not be biologically cured, a spiritual healing takes place. Therefore, while cure is not always possible, there is always room for healing. Healing can be experienced as acceptance of illness and being at peace with one's life. Healing, at its core, is spiritual (Puchalski 2001a).

What is Spirituality, Then?

M. Downey defines spirituality as: 'An awareness that there are levels of reality not immediately apparent and that there is a quest for personal integration in the face of forces of fragmentation and depersonalization' (1997: 14). Puchalski provides a relatively simple definition of spirituality as 'that aspect of human beings that seeks to heal or to be whole' (2001b). Spirituality, then, is not synonymous with religion, but is something more vast, and includes — besides the beliefs — the culture, the taboos, the practices (yoga and meditation), and the lifestyle of an individual — his interaction with the cosmos around.

Role of Spirituality in Health: Where is the Evidence?

The healthcare community and the public at large have become increasingly interested in the relationship between spirituality and health. However, many clinicians remain sceptical of spirituality; they are uncomfortable discussing it, and are unsure about how to respond to, or how to incorporate, spirituality into their practices (Droege 1991). Engaging patients in a dialogue about spiritual needs can result in an enriching, enlightening and rewarding experience, for not only the patients, but also the physicians. But an objective mind would then ask, 'Where is the evidence for such thinking?'

Several national surveys, including the Gallup polls (1990, 1997), showed that patients do want their spiritual concerns to be addressed by their physicians (Gallup 1990). The studies looking into the role of spirituality in health, and the benefits thereof, can be largely grouped under the following four headings:

Mortality

W. J. Strawbridge et al., in a peer-reviewed study (1997), showed that people who followed regular spiritual practices lived longer. A scientific mechanism for this difference was also put forward: Interleukin-6, which is a mediator for many illnesses in the body, was much less elevated in those who attended church than in non-churchgoers (Koenig et al. 1997).

Coping

Spirituality helps in coping with illness, pain, and the stresses of life. Spiritual practitioners have a more positive outlook and a better quality of life, even in diseased states. Advanced cancer patients found comfort in their religious and spiritual beliefs, were happier, more satisfied with life, and felt less pain (Yates et al. 1981). Brady et al. suggested that spiritual wellbeing was related to the ability to enjoy life, even in the midst of symptoms, including pain, and therefore spirituality may in fact be an important clinical target (1999). The results of the pain questionnaire distributed by the American Pain Society to hospitalised patients showed that personal prayer was the most commonly used non-drug method of controlling pain, with 76 per cent of the patients making use of it (McNeill et al. 1998).

Recovery

Spiritual commitments also enhance recovery from any illness. A study of heart transplant patients showed that those who participated in religious activities complied better with follow-up treatment, had improved physical functioning at the 12-month follow-up, had higher levels of self-esteem, and had less anxiety and fewer health worries (Harris et al. 1995). Spirituality also enables people to worry less and thus reduce stress. Going hand-in-hand with spirituality is the power of 'hope and positive thinking', which may in fact have a placebo effect on disease and illness. If our beliefs are powerful, they can influence our health outcomes (Beecher 1955). H. Benson, a cardiologist at Harvard School of Medicine, describes this placebo effect as 'remembered wellness — an ability to tap into one's inner resources to heal' (Puchalski 2001a: 354).

The doctor–patient relationship in fact itself has a placebo effect, and therefore, it is not only the spirituality of the patient, but also that of the doctor that matters. There is an objective basis to all these actions of spirituality, as demonstrated by Benson during his research in the 1960s, when he showed that transcendental meditation for 10–20 minutes twice a day led to decreased metabolism, heart rate, respiratory rate, and slower brain waves. The practice was beneficial in the treatment of chronic pains, insomnia, anxiety, depression, premenstrual syndromes, infertility, cancers, HIV, and in end-of-life issues. In fact, Benson concluded, 'To the extent that any disease is caused or made worse by stress, to that extent, evoking the relaxation response is an effective therapy' (2001). Stress has become such an integral part of our modern lifestyle that almost 60–90 per cent of patients visiting a physician may have diseases related to stress, like high blood pressure, headache, and irritable bowel syndrome. Indeed, virtually, stress is a component — if not causative, then certainly incremental — for most diseases.

End-of-life issues

End-of-life issues, too, find comfort in spirituality. When asked what helped them cope with their gynaecological cancer, 93 per cent out of 108 women cited spiritual beliefs (Roberts et al. 1997). Similarly, among 90 HIV-positive patients, those who were spiritually active had less fear of death and less guilt (Kaldjian et al. 1998). In a random Gallup poll, when a general demographic was asked what concerns they would have if they were dying, their foremost concerns turned out to be companionship and spiritual comfort (George H. Gallup International Institute et al. 1997).

Presenting path-breaking research at the Heart Failure Society of America in 2006, Dr Patricia Uber from the University of Maryland, Baltimore, commented that the breathing pattern alters in heart failure, and that breath becomes increasingly out of synchrony with blood pressure oscillations (cited in Wood 2006). *Pranayam* helps restore the respiratory cycle to the Mayer Wave oscillations, and harmonises blood pressure and breathing. Uber further presented data from studies showing that recitation of the rosary (in Latin) or yogic mantras can reduce the frequency of breath, respiratory variability, and baro reflex sensitivity. Even volitional breathing, wherein the breath is slowed to a rate of six breaths per minute, practised for one hour daily over a period of one month, reduced the breathing rate, increased VO_2 Max and the anaerobic threshold (ibid.). In fact, in some studies the improvement seen in baro reflex sensitivity with deep breathing was equal to that seen with long-term drug therapy. So therapies that reduce neuro-hormonal levels, stress levels, blood pressure, and heart rate without use of a device or a gamut of drugs, instead involving simple practices such as meditation, rhythmic breathing exercises, going to religious places, etc., may go a long way in providing succour to terminally ill patients. This has even more relevance in developing and financially impoverished countries like ours. As Dr Patricia Uber commented — 'it's time we start addressing complimentary medicine, for we would really be crazy to just keep stacking on neuro-hormonal antagonism and devices without even looking at the mind–body connection' (ibid.).

Relevance of Spirituality

Understanding patient spirituality in the context of healthcare delivery is extremely important for many reasons:

1. Spirituality may be a dynamic variable in the patient's understanding of the disease. An example is the belief in the most

remote corners of our country that diseases are caused by the wrath of god.

2. Religious convictions may affect decision-making in health care. An example of this would be the rejection of blood transfusion by Jehovah's Witnesses, a millenarian Christian denomination.[1]
3. Spirituality may be a patient need and may be important in helping patients to cope with the disease, and to find meaning behind disease, suffering and death.
4. An understanding of the patient's spirituality is integral to holistic patient care and in healing the patient, as against a technical fix or a mechanical cure.
5. Spirituality helps in end-of-life issues by providing a meaning to death and in developing a partnership with God.
6. Spirituality does have a negative influence at times and sometimes an individual's belief may work against his self, but again, the study of spirituality would help in coping with these negative influences (Puchalski 2001a).

Do Patients Want Spirituality?

The answer is a categorical 'Yes!' In fact, after the 1997 poll, George H. Gallup Jr. wrote, 'the over-arching message that emerges from this study is that the American people want to reclaim and reassert the spiritual dimensions in dying' (George H. Gallup International Institute et al. 1997). In a previous 1990 Gallup survey, 75 per cent of Americans had opined that religion was central to their lives, and a majority felt that their spiritual faiths could help them recover from their illnesses (Gallup 1990). In a 1996 *USA Today Weekend* Health Survey, 63 per cent of the patients surveyed believed that it is good for doctors to talk to patients about spiritual beliefs (McNichol 1996). Similarly, Ehman and colleagues found that in their survey, 68 per cent of patients said they would welcome a spiritual question in a medical history, while 15 per cent said they actually recalled being asked by the physicians whether spiritual and religious beliefs would influence their decisions (Ehman et al. 1999). These figures are likely to be much higher in our country. But unfortunately, spirituality has been virtually eliminated and long overlooked in our medical school curricula and in the standards of medical care. It is urgent that we restore an engagement with, and awareness of, spirituality in all these arenas.

The Science of Spirituality

Traditionally, the body has been considered a composite of the physical body and the 'vital body'; it includes the 'soul' or the 'spirit'. The physical body is like computer hardware, in which the vital body acts like software. It is not only the physical body, but also the vital body that has a quantum nature (Goswami 2004/2005). The Eastern system of medicine has concentrated on healing the vital body under the belief that it is the root cause of most illnesses, and the corollary of healing it, is healing the physical body as well. The Western system of medicine has focused mainly on the physical body. Both these systems are good and have their place, but as Dr A. Goswami from the Department of Physics and the Institute of Theoretical Science, University of Oregon, says, 'Both systems of medicine are very good at what they do, but alone neither is the perfect apple of holistic health that holds the key to all cures' (ibid.). He further attempts to integrate the two sciences through 'science within consciousness', which he proposes on the basis of quantum physics. What is lacking in the field of mind–body medicine is a clear understanding of the mechanism by which mind and body can interact, and where the causal efficacy of that interaction lies. The absence of this understanding impedes progress in the field. The Eastern philosophy of medicine (alternative medicine) uses such concepts as the flow of *Chi* (*Ki* in Japan) or *Prana* in healing practices. The corresponding concept used in alternative medicine in the West is that of 'vital energy'. But in all these practices, the causal role of consciousness is ignored. We therefore need a new integrated science of health and healing which recognises and incorporates the role of consciousness in health and disease (Puchalski 2004). It is here that quantum physics provides objectivity to what has been known and preached even in our ancient scriptures. Quantum physics propounds that matter and object exist as waves of possibility and probability that can be present at any one moment in time at two or more places. Further, in addition to a continuous movement of a wave form, particles can also have discontinuous quantum leaps, and there can be non-local interactions in addition to local ones. These quantum possibility waves collapse to 'actuality' through the mechanics of measurement. So, in reality, consciousness is the transcendent ground of being, and we must see matter as quantum possibility waves within it (Goswami 2004/2005).

This raises the question: Is consciousness due to the brain? The answer lies in the concept of 'tangled hierarchy'. Take the example of the liar's paradox. If a liar says, 'I am a liar', it is a tangled hierarchy because the predicate qualifies the subject; however, the subject too qualifies the predicate. If a liar says, 'I am a liar', he is telling the truth; in which case, his saying that he is a liar is a lie, and so on, ad infinitum. This tangle, according to Dr Goswami, can be seen and resolved only by 'jumping out of the system, but we cannot see it, if we identify with the system' (2004/2005: 47–48). The same can be said about the tangled hierarchy between consciousness and the brain. A decapitated person cannot make any quantum measurements, but by the same token, without consciousness, the brain too cannot make any measurements. So there is a circularity here — without brain awareness, there is no consciousness; but without consciousness, there is no unique brain state of awareness either. The resolution of this circularity lies in the concept of 'dependant co-arising' in quantum physics. Here, the brain's awareness of the object and consciousness co-create each other, that too simultaneously.

Similarly, the mind is not the same as the brain, and that being so, one needs to find a mediator for the interaction between the mind and the brain. In this quest, University of Mexico neurophysiologists Grinberg-Zylberbaum et al. conducted a simple, yet ingenious, experiment to demonstrate quantum non-local connection between human brains. Two subjects were asked to meditate for about 20 minutes with the intent of establishing direct communication. They were then put in separate Faraday chambers, which were electro-magnetically isolated enclosures, while maintaining their direct communication, and their brain waves (EEG) were recorded. When the first subject was shown a series of light flashes, his brain responded with electrical activity, called the evoked potentials. Surprisingly, the second subject's brain, which received no stimulus, also exhibited electrical activity of similar phase and strength on its EEG, called transferred potentials (Zylberbaum et al. 1994). This brings us to the question of what caused the first person's evoked potentials to create the second person's transferred potentials. And the answer is — consciousness. Since there was no material interaction, it was only through non-local communicating attributes of consciousness that the contact could be maintained. So the model that emerges shows that ultimately, there is only consciousness; that there is no manifest 'physical body' or any manifest 'mental body' and no dualism; that the physical and the mental body are embedded in a transcendent consciousness as mere possibilities. It is with this realisation and the objective and scientific basis provided by quantum physics that a new science of healing, called mind–body healing, is emerging. However, the Western system of medicine is reluctant to accept it because of the dualism of mind and body perceived by them in this system.

Consciousness is such a blissful mediator that the element of dualism is totally negated. Therefore, mind–body healing is nothing but quantum healing — an idea that has already been creatively intuited by a number of medical practitioners, especially L. Dossey and D. Chopra.

> The puzzle of mind–body healing is, how a thought, a non-material object, can cause the brain to make a material object, a neuro-peptide molecule, for example, that will initiate a communication to the immune or the endocrine system, eventually leading to healing (Goswami 2004/2005: 47–48).

In fact, Dossey has worked on the non-locality of this quantum healing, and his point is further proved by a study by R. C. Byrd involving 393 patients at the San Francisco General Hospital's Cardiac Care Unit, on the effect of prayers on their recovery offered remotely by home prayer groups. The prayed-for patients were five times less likely to require antibiotics and three times less prone to develop fluid in the lungs than those for whom prayers had not been offered. So when somebody prays for an ailing person at a distance, consciousness simultaneously absorbs the healing thought in the mind, as in mental telepathy, although the patient may not be aware of it (because of noise and other events occurring in the mind–brain complex). This in turn leads to quantum healing, as it occurs in self-healing (Goswami 2004/2005).

In the Chinese system of medicine, the vital energy or *Chi* flows along certain pre-defined pathways called 'meridians', and these are used as acupuncture or acupressure points. Similarly, in ancient Indian and Ayurvedic systems of medicine, the vital energy, known as *Prana*, is mapped along pathways called *naadi*s. Although these *naadi*s do not coincide with the Chinese meridians, there are similarities. The energy in the Chinese system of medicine has two complementary aspects, called Yin and Yang, and it is the balance between Yin and Yang which determines the health of an individual.

The concept of vital energy was discarded in Western philosophy and biology because of the advent of molecular biology, where anything and everything could be explained at the level of DNA. But DNA alone cannot explain mind–body healing. Molecules obey physical laws, but they know nothing about the context of living, such as maintenance and survival, let alone love or jealousy, that preoccupies us for much of our lives (Goswami 2004/2005).

Is it possible to feel somebody else's emotions? Yes, it is possible to do so through quantum non-locality of the vital body, which is akin to mental telepathy, and is called empathy. Using the same quantum non-locality, it is possible for a person of healthy *Chi* or *Prana* to help another person balance his or her *Chi* or *Prana*.

Mind–Body Healing: Practical Model

Our body already has, in many cases of illnesses, the required and requisite wisdom and mechanisms for cure. We just have to discover it and manifest it (Moss 1981). To discover this hidden talent of the body to heal itself, we need to go through four stages of creativity, viz., preparation, incubation, insight, and manifestation with understanding (Goswami 2004/2005).

In the first step of preparation, the patient should be encouraged to research the disease and meditate on it. This will readily show the role of mental stress in disease causation and the root cause of mental stress accumulation will also become clear, which is mental speed — hurrying and rushing about — and augmenting the pursuit of desires with anxieties and day-dreams (ibid.). So the purpose of the preparatory stage is to slow down the mind, and to create an open and receptive mind, which is an essential requisite for creativity. The second stage is that of unconscious processing, where we use unlearned stimuli to generate uncollapsed possibility waves, but we do not choose, because choosing will involve conscious awareness (Moss 1984). The third process of insight involves mental visualisation and imagination of healing and the power of positive thinking, which triggers the corrective vital body movements. As for the final phase of manifestation, once healing has occurred, the patient must bring to manifestation some of the lifestyle changes that were intuited during the creative insight phase, if they want the remission to be stable and permanent. The Western system of medicine aspires to correct the physical body by the brute force of chemistry, radiation, surgery, medicine, and so on. But a more creative approach would use the mental body, mental imagination and visualisation to try to trigger the correct vital body movement, which corrects the physical body's aberrations. For such creative healing to occur, however, there is a need for a change in the role and behavioural patterns of physicians, from a hierarchical, dominant and authoritarian positioning closer to that of a partner sharing experiences, a co-learning relationship — a tangled hierarchy (Goswami 2004/2005).

How Do We Propagate Spirituality in Health?

The first step would be accepting spirituality as an integral component of healthcare delivery and giving it national recognition. This has already taken place overseas, but unfortunately India, a country of sages, saints and faith healers, the very cradle of spirituality in fact, is only beginning to take small steps towards such a change. The Joint Commission on Accreditation of Health Care Organizations in USA states, 'For many patients pastoral care and other spiritual services are an integral part of health care in daily life. The hospital is able to provide for pastoral care and other spiritual services for the patients who request them' (Puchalski 2001a: 355). The American College of Physicians also recognised the role of spirituality and in an end-of-life consensus panel, opined, 'Physicians should extend the care for those with serious medical illness by attention to psycho-social, existential or spiritual suffering' (ibid.). In 1992, only three medical schools in America offered courses on Spirituality and Health, while in 2001, 75 out of a total of 125 schools were offering these courses (ibid.). In fact, the Association of American Medical Colleges convened a consensus group of Deans and faculty of medical schools to determine the key elements of medical school curricula (Lo et al. 1999). In its first report, it listed the essential attributes of physicians. The first attribute is that the physician should be altruistic:

> Physicians must be compassionate and empathetic in caring for patients . . . In all of their interactions with patients, they must seek to understand the meaning of the patients' stories in the context of the patients' beliefs and family and cultural values . . . They must continue to care for dying patients even when disease specific therapy is no longer available or desired (ibid.).

In fact, in the George Washington University School of Medicine, spirituality is interwoven with the rest of the curricula throughout the four years of medical school, so that students learn to integrate it into all of their practices (Puchalski 2001a).

In its policy statement, the Association of American Medical Colleges acknowledges the role of spirituality in health, and states,

> [s]pirituality is recognized as a factor that contributes to health in many persons. The concept of spirituality is found in all cultures and societies. It is expressed in an individual's search for ultimate meaning through participation in religion and/or belief in God, family, naturalism, rationalism, humanism and the arts. All of these factors can influence how patients and health care professionals perceive health and illness and how they interact with one another (1998).

It is therefore crucial that spirituality be a subject, as important as others, in our medical school curricula, and in fact should also be included in school curricula, as the formative years of life develop our spiritual beliefs and practices, which may be difficult to change in later years.

Sceptic's Viewpoint

Even if spirituality plays a role in health matters, questions persist about whether physicians should encourage religious and spiritual practices, and if so, what should be the role of the chaplain, clergy, priests, and pandits? Also, there are concerns about whether the physician should guide or lead in spirituality. In such a case, would the physician's personal faith and beliefs influence a patient who may be very vulnerable at that moment in time? Would it lead to proselytising? Where are the boundaries, therefore, between what physicians do and what should be left to the priesthood (Sloan et al. 2000)? It is important to note that because physicians are not trained to engage in in-depth discussions with patients about spiritual concerns, patients seeking spiritual support should be referred to a chaplain or other clergy. However, Puchalski disagrees with this stance, and believes that a physician can work together with a chaplain, and that physicians should be trained to respond in an appropriate manner to any spiritual inquiry or take into consideration an individual's spiritual history. She further adds, '[a]n agnostic patient should not be told to engage in worship any more than a highly religious patient should be criticized for frequent church attendance. Proselytizing is never appropriate in a clinical setting' (2001b: 34).

The spiritual issues that one faces in the day-to-day practice of medicine and in day-to-day life are those associated with acute and chronic illnesses, and include meaninglessness, hopelessness, despair, lack of forgiveness, abandonment, anger, and the feeling of being unloved or unconnected (Droege 1991). Spiritual care is inter-disciplinary, and a physician's attention to the spiritual needs of a patient is not intended to replace the priesthood and other faith-based professionals, but rather to complement the role they may play in alleviating a patient's suffering. This integration of spirituality in healthcare delivery should not be coercive, but doctor-initiated and patient-dictated.

Conclusion

The medical profession should very seriously, and sooner rather than later, rediscover and reinvent the role of spirituality in every patient's wellbeing in the holistic sense. Spirituality is as much the root cause of disease as bacteria and viruses. A doctor has an important role in exploring the role of spirituality in an individual's disease process, and then helping to ameliorate and heal the patient as a whole, rather than attempting to cure just the physical body. Physicians, by recognising the spiritual dimensions of their professional lives, can reclaim the spiritual roots of their practice, viz., compassion and service. They can also restore the art of the practice of medicine to the science of medicine, in the process restoring the medical profession to the pedestal of godliness, which it has occupied since time immemorial.

So what we need is not to decry either the Western system of medicine or the Eastern, but to integrate both of them. The Western philosophy of the physical body chemistry is important as the hardware of the computer, but equally important are the software components, viz., the vital body movements and consciousness. The wellbeing and wholeness of the body requires a homeostasis between both elements.

Note

1. Jehovah's Witnesses reject blood transfusion, even in emergencies, on the grounds that the Bible prohibits the ingestion of blood. See http://www.afn.org/~afn52344/dissertation1.html (accessed 14 September 2011) for a comprehensive discussion of the medical and legal complexities involved in the matter.

References

Association of American Medical Colleges. 1998. 'Report I: Learning Objectives for Medical Student Education: Guidelines for Medical Schools', Medical School Objectives Project. Washington, DC: American Association of Medical Colleges. Available at https://members.aamc.org/eweb/upload/Learning%20Objectives%20for%20Medical%20Student%20Educ%20Report%20I.pdf (accessed 2 April 2013).

———. 1999. 'Report III: Contemporary Issues in Medicine: Communication in Medicine', Medical School Objectives Project. Washington, DC: Association of American Medical Colleges. Available at https://members.aamc.org/eweb/upload/Contemporary%20Issues%20In%20Med%20Commun%20in%20Medicine%20Report%20III%20.pdf (accessed 2 April 2013).

Beecher, H. K. 1955. 'The Powerful Placebo', *Journal of the American Medical Association*, 159 (17): 1602–06.

Benson, H. 1990. *The Relaxation Response*. New York: Avon.

———. 1996. *Timeless Healing: The Power and Biology of Belief.* New York: Simon and Schuster.

———. 2001. 'Spirituality and Healing in Medicine: Introduction', *Harvard Medical School: Department of Continuing Education*. Available at http://cme.hms.harvard.edu/syllabi.asp?task=benson (accessed 2 April 2013).

Brady, M. J., A. H. Peterman, G. Fitchett, M. Mo, and D. Cella. 1999. 'A Case for Including Spirituality in Quality of Life Measurement in Oncology', *Psycho-Oncology*, 8 (5): 417–28.

Byrd, R. C. 1988. 'Positive Therapeutic Effects of Intercessory Prayer in a Coronary Care Unit Population', *Southern Medical Journal*, 81: 826–29.

Cassell, E. J. 2003. *The Nature of Suffering and Goals of Medicine*. New York: Oxford University Press.

Chopra, D. 1990. *Quantum Healing: Exploring the Frontiers of Mind/Body Medicine*. New York: Bantam Books.

Dossey, L. 1989. *Recovering the Soul: A Scientific and Spiritual Search*. New York: Bantam Books.

Downey, M. 1997. *Understanding Christian Spirituality*. Mahwah, NJ: Paulist Press.

Droege, T. A. 1991. *The Faith Factor in Healing*. Philadelphia: Trinity Press.

Ehman, J. W., B. B. Ott, T. H. Short, R. C. Ciampa, and J. Hansen-Flaschen. 1999. 'Do Patients Want Physicians to Inquire about Their Spiritual Or Religious Beliefs If They Become Gravely Ill?', *Archives of Internal Medicine*, 159 (15): 1803–06.

Frankl, V. E. 1984. *Man's Search for Meaning*. New York: Simon and Schuster.

Gallup, G. 1990. *Religion in America 1990: The Gallup Opinion Index 1979–80*. Princeton, NJ: Princeton Religion and Research Center.

George H. Gallup International Institute, Nathan Cummings Foundation and Fetzer Institute. 1997. *Spiritual Beliefs and the Dying Process: A Report on a National Survey*. Princeton, NJ: George H. Gallup International Institute.

Goswami, A. 2004/2005. 'Quantum Physics, Consciousness and a New Science of Mind-Body Healing', *Savijnanam: Journal of the Bhaktivedanta Institute*, 3–4: 47–48.

———. 1993. *The Self-Aware Universe: How Consciousness Creates the Material World*. New York: Tarcher, Putnam.

Grinberg-Zylberbaum, J., M. Delaflor, L. Attie, et al. 1994. 'Einstein-Podolsky-Rosen Paradox in the Human Brain: The Transferred Potential', *Physics Essays*, 7: 422–28.

Harris, R. C., M. A. Dew, A. Lee, et al. 1995. 'The Role of Religion in Heart Transplant Recipient's Long Term Health and Well Being', *Journal of Religion and Health*, 34 (1): 17–32.

Joint Commission on Accreditation of Healthcare Organisations (JCAHO). 1999. 'Patient Rights and Organization Ethics', in JCAHO, *Comprehensive Accreditation Manual for Hospitals (CAMH): The Official Handbook (Update 3)*. Oakbrook Terrace, III: JCAHO.

Kaldjian, L. C., J. F. Jekel and G. Friedland. 1998. 'End-of-life Decisions in HIV Positive Patients: The Role of Spiritual Beliefs', *AIDS*, 12 (1): 103–07.

Koenig, H. G., H. J. Cohen, L. K. George, J. C. Hays, D. B. Larson, and D. G. Blazer. 1997. 'Attendance at Religious Services, Interleukin-6, and Other Biological Parameters of Immune Function in Older Adults', *International Journal of Psychiatry in Medicine*, 27 (3): 233–50.

Lo, B., T. Quill, T. Tulsky, The ACP-ASIM End-of-Life Care Consensus Panel. 1999. 'Discussing Palliative Care with Patients', *Annals of Internal Medicine*, 130 (9): 744–49.

McNeill, J. A., G. D. Sherwood, P. L. Starck, and C. J. Thompson. 1998. 'Assessing Clinical Outcomes: Patient Satisfaction with Pain Management', *Journal of Pain and Symptom Management*, 16 (1): 29–40.

McNichol, T. 1996. 'The New Faith in Medicine', *USA Today Weekend*, 5–7 April: 4–5. (Survey conducted February 1996 by ICR Research Group).

Moss, R. 1981. *The I That Is We*. Berkeley CA: Celestial Arts.

———. 1984. *Radical Aliveness*. Berkeley CA: Celestial Arts.

Puchalski, C. M. 2001a. 'The Role of Spirituality in Health Care', *Proceedings* (*Baylor University Medical Centre*), 14 (4): 352–57.

———. 2001b. 'Spirituality and Health: The Art of Compassionate Medicine', *Hospital Physician*, 37 (3): 30–40.

———. 2004. 'Spirituality and Health: Implications for Clinical Practice'. Paper presented at CME, sponsored by The New York Academy of Medicine and the HIP Health Plan at New York, 2 December.

Roberts, J. A., D. Brown, T. Elkins, and D. B. Larson. 1997. 'Factors Influencing View of Patients with Gynaecologic Cancer about End-of-Life Decisions', *American Journal of Obstetrics and Gynecology*, 176 (1/1): 166–72.

Sloan, R. P., E. Bagiella, L. VandeCreek, M. Hover, C. Casalone, Jinpu Hirsch, T. Y. Hasan, R. Kreger, and P. Poulos. 2000. 'Should Physicians Prescribe Religious Activities?', *New England Journal of Medicine*, 342 (25): 1913–16.

Strawbridge, W. J., R. D. Cohen, S. J. Shema, et al. 1997. 'Frequent Attendance at Religious Services and Mortality over 28 Years', *American Journal of Public Health*, 87: 957–61.

Wood, Shelley. 2006. 'Poetry, Prayers and *Pranayam*: A Low Tech Therapy for Heart Failure', *HeartWire*, 13 September. Available at http://www.theheart.org/article/741763.do (accessed 2 April 2013).

Yates, J. W., B. J. Chalmer, St. James P., M. Follansbee, and F. P. McKegney. 1981. 'Religion in Patients with Advanced Cancer', *Medical and Paediatric Oncology*, 9 (2): 121–28.

Four

Healing Minds and Bodies

What Place for Spirituality?

Roger Worthington

Healing works at different levels and medical science can explain some, but not all, of the mechanisms involved. Spiritual aspects of human healing are necessarily difficult to explain, and at best what can be explained is how scientific and spiritual accounts of healing inter-relate. Exploring these relations properly requires the reader to call into question the *nature* of mind and consciousness, including necessary distinctions between mind and body. These ideas, which some regard as controversial, are to be found embedded deep within Himalayan thought and spiritual tradition. Western accounts of science and healing tend to take a different approach, partly because of unease about what is termed 'dualism', and partly because of scepticism about spirituality itself. Bridging these gaps presents serious difficulties, but the attempt is nonetheless worth making.

Minds and bodies are part of an integrated whole, and if, as sometimes happens, bodies do not heal in the way that they should, there may be purely physical (medical) explanations for why this is. An alternative explanation might be that the underlying causes are reflective of a state of mind, and lack of equilibrium or general well-being. By this account, if 'lack of union' is the root cause of illness or non-healing, then questions arise as to what the best remedies to try and restore wholeness are, and the best course of action to take to help prevent problems in the future. The aim of this chapter is not to look at mechanisms, but rather to look for answers by exploring relationships between 'healer', 'healing', and 'the healed' within a broad context of science and spiritual philosophy.

A Rationale

Many things in life can be explained by the application of a logical scientific method, but in general, healing is not one of them. Healing has an element of mystery, but this need not imply that attempts at rational explanation will necessarily prove futile. If there is no apparent explanation for *how* something comes about, it is possibly an indication that the wrong vocabulary or the wrong tools are being used in the analysis. While scientific explanations exist to describe mechanisms for *how* the human body heals, in no way do these exclude other (that is, spiritual) dimensions to healing. This is especially so if the causes of not being *whole* (literally, non-healing) lie deep within the *nature* of the person, as opposed to in ordinary physical mechanisms that govern the human body. Separating the two aspects of healing — the side that is rational and scientific, and the side that does not lend itself to empirical observation — is a mistake, and the one should be regarded as being integral to the other.

Healing

It can generally be acknowledged that medicine is not a complete science, and that uncertainty is an ever-present reality. Healing, on the other hand, is about restoring wholeness in the person, not applications of bio-medical science. According to Himalayan traditions, for patients to heal fully, they should strive to depend upon themselves as much as — or more than — on the physician (except perhaps on occasions when a patient is too sick, when dependence becomes inevitable). Promoting effective healing makes demands on the patient as well as on the physician, both of whom can benefit from developing awareness of the inner dimensions that exist to healing. Attitudes as well as attributes contribute to the healing process, that is, by means of the therapeutic relationship and the application of skill or 'techne'. Being in possession of requisite technical knowledge and skill can enable someone to become a physician; however, it is much less clear what makes someone a healer, or for that matter, *how* someone comes to be healed.

In the case of a physician, knowledge, skill and experience can be acquired by study, hard work, and by the practice of medicine itself. However, in the case of a *healer* there is no clear method of acquisition, since inner personal attributes play the major part. While these are a matter of someone's inner characteristics, they too can be acquired, for example, by pursuit of a path of self-discipline. Such are the Himalayan teachings, including those associated with the practice of *Raja Yoga*. Fundamentally, healer and healed should be seen as participants in a unified process of healing.

Raja Yoga and Modern Medicine

The term literally means 'kingly yoga'. In that yoga means 'union', 'kingly union' is effectively a path that encompasses all other categories or schools of yoga — hence its pre-eminent status.[1] *Raja yoga* is difficult to follow and generally requires a teacher or guru. Therefore, it is not for everyone, and is unlikely ever to be accepted by a wide body of opinion, regardless of cultural or religious background. It is being discussed here because it can help to unlock at least some of the mysteries of healing, mainly by virtue of offering rational explanations for the phenomenon known as 'consciousness'. Without understanding more about consciousness, it will never be possible to understand the mechanisms of healing.

Engagement in the healing process is most often inward and may not be verbally articulated, which raises the interesting question of whether or not a patient has to believe in a form of healing in order for it to work. The answer is probably 'no', although in the absence of belief it is perhaps unlikely that somebody would seek out such a healer. Belief is not directly part of the healing process, and if it were, then reliance on belief would necessarily exclude those who do not hold the 'right' belief. Healers who practice therapies such as Reiki or Ayurvedic medicine might need to believe in what they themselves are doing more than other practitioners (for example, of modern allopathic medicine), but that belief does not necessarily have to be shared by their patients. If spirituality is part of an inner process that can help enable and promote healing, it neither implies that science should be discarded, nor that religion is the only thing capable of playing a part in the process of healing.

Religion is too often busy with ritual observance, organisations and rules, any or all of which can become a hindrance in terms of facilitating inward reflection. Religion and spirituality can go together, and it was long assumed that one did not exist without the other; however, history and experience would suggest otherwise. Spirituality is a state of union between inner and outer aspects of the self, and this union is what fundamentally enables healing to take place. Although modern allopathic medicine tends to be something applied *to* or practised *on* a patient, it is perfectly possible for scientific knowledge to be employed to help promote healing as a restoration of wholeness. If promoting wellbeing for healer and healed strengthens their relationship, this in turn helps to restore connections between doctor and patient, which are often relatively weak in modern medical practice.

The interaction between physician–healer and patient takes place on many different levels, and it should not be seen as being restricted to the administration of medicine or to any form of physical intervention. The physician can function as a facilitator or enabler of healing, but physicians often view healing with scepticism, and at first sight it does not sit comfortably with the scientific model. However, this need not necessarily be the case, and there is nothing stopping a healer-physician from consciously or unconsciously drawing on his/her inner spiritual strength. Himalayan traditions recognise that there is both a spiritual and a scientific side to healing. In general, awareness of this is something that comes about through sustained effort, such as following a path of yoga over time.

The practice of medicine is a shared enterprise in which physician and patient both play a role. If the reader is able and willing to acknowledge that there is a spiritual dimension to healing, then medicine and healing can reasonably co-exist; and if that position is accepted, the apparent dichotomy between scientific and spiritual explanations for healing turn out to be false. The best results ultimately come about when there is a state of union between the healer, the one who is healed, and the process of healing, whether or not this state of union is consciously experienced.

Modern technologies have great investigative powers, upon which physicians have come to depend, and patients themselves have become used to these technological interventions. However, medicine is weakened if it becomes wholly dependent upon practical applications of modern science and technology. True healing is something much more sophisticated than mere technological application; it is both a science and an art. That is the source of its strength, and if healer, the healed, and the act of healing are all one, this effectively mirrors the state of union that is said to exist between the knower, the known, and the act of knowing described in the *Yoga Sutras*.[2]

Teachings from the *rishis* or spiritual teachers, which are not normally written down but rather handed down by oral tradition, point to the reversal between what is perceived as 'real' and what *is* 'real' — that is, pure essence devoid of any gross material form. No empirical evidence can be marshalled in support of this explanation; none is ever possible. But there is a long tradition that supports this line of reasoning, including, for example, that contained within the *Ashtanga* or eight-limbed school of yoga. This is the other name for *Raja Yoga*, which Patanjali codified in his famous aphorisms.

Patanjali left a systematic account of daily discipline, whereby there is a bringing together of the conscious thinking mind and the higher principle, known as 'mind' (or, in Sanskrit, simply *manas*, which has no real equivalence in English). It is at this level that real discoveries can be made, and it is with regard to mind and consciousness that Eastern and Western approaches to healing are most at variance with one another.

Minds and Bodies

The unity of existence does not permit artificial distinctions. Science and spirituality are part of a whole in the same way that mind and body are part of a whole. Just as science does not exist in a vacuum, spirituality is an aspect of human existence that touches every domain, including (but not limited to) science and scientific knowledge. The *Yoga Sutra*s define ignorance as a form of illusion, the Sanskrit term *avidya* (illusion) meaning 'not-knowing' or 'lack of wisdom'. Disconnection or *dis* unity between mind and body is essentially harmful to wellbeing, and lack of awareness of the inner nature of existence, as outlined in the *Sutra*s, is clearly identified as a root cause of suffering.[3]

According to Patanjali, the opposite of 'not-knowing' is *vidya* (wisdom), which is inner or spiritual knowing. Interestingly, this same term is sometimes used to describe scientific or technical knowledge. Context and application determine which meaning is applicable, and while much human effort goes into the scientific form of knowing, very little normally goes into the spiritual type of knowing. It could even be said that the pursuit of inner knowledge is the purpose of all existence; therefore, failing to acknowledge the importance of inner knowledge is in a sense to deny the true nature of the self.

Himalayan teachings hold that mind and brain are different in the way they operate, having different modes of operation and characteristic properties. Mind, according to these teachings, is a universal principle. It is not particular to the individual, and it finds expression through (but is not synonymous with) the physical organ of the human brain. To say that mind and brain are part of a whole is different from saying that they are one and the same, and although it is not possible to divide a unity, it is possible to have two or more parts of a whole.

To confuse mind and brain, or to have them the wrong way round, suggesting that brain function determines how the mind works, is not helpful, in spite of the fact that mind and brain clearly interconnect. Mind, like spirit (but unlike the brain), is not confined to the physical body; it is universal, not particular, and so at a higher level it is shared with others, whether or not the connections are perceived. This may seem an extraordinary proposition, especially given how attached people are to their thoughts and ideas most of the time. However, that does not make this rationale wrong. Science needs a method for dealing with the unseen side of existence, and this is the level at which interconnections between seen and unseen really work.

In the past, various explanations were offered to try to explain the unseen elements in nature, and while science may be regarded as inextricably bound to the material world, that is not always the case, and not all existence is so comprised in terms of hard matter. In short, science needs a way to deal with the *im*material world, and giving recognition to the spiritual dimension of human existence is one way of achieving this goal. Scientific knowledge and inner knowledge are not necessarily opposites, and the perceived disjunction between the two types of knowledge is really a form of illusion. Bringing them back together again is effectively what is really meant by speaking about the unity of existence.

Mind has a creative energy that channels itself through the brain, but not all brain function is creative. Some of it is concerned with performing tasks such as breathing, digestion and locomotion, which require little or no conscious effort. While deliberate use of the brain can enable a person to perform complex, creative tasks, this is a different exercise, and here it is 'mind' that is really in charge. One could ask, 'How can the brain ask itself anything because that suggests that the brain itself is split', but the inference is not justified. Thought is intrinsic to the brain, and it is both logical and possible for the 'brain' to think about itself — if and only if 'mind' is accorded its proper place.

If it is accepted that the brain controls body function and that mind controls the brain, then it is not a leap of faith to suggest that bringing mind, brain and body into alignment will help promote healing. If a physician helps bring this about so much the better, but it can happen without outside intervention if the individual is able to achieve this 'alignment' by the exercise or application of inner discipline. Mind is never 'owned'; it is attributed to 'persons', but the connection is not physical. The organ 'brain' is, however, physical, being always and in every way particular to the individual. Thought originates in the mind and finds expression through being processed by the brain, and it is this relationship that is so central to ancient Himalayan teachings about mind and consciousness.

However, this is not in accord with Western analytic traditions that tend to conflate mind with brain, which is to commit a category error — one to which people have so long grown accustomed that they are not even aware of the error. Descartes assigned to 'spirit' or 'ether' that which was not visible or capable of rational explanation and material proof. But by separating matter from spirit, the body assumes a largely mechanistic role, thereby making the charge of 'dualism' levelled by philosophers more difficult to defend. With Descartes' body and spirit, one imbues the other, but this overlooks the fact that they are really part of an integrated whole, and overall, his explanations are perhaps more incomplete than fundamentally 'wrong'.

While in ordinary waking consciousness mind works in close affinity with the brain, in sleep and in deeper levels of consciousness the association is much looser, making it impossible for mind to be contained within, or defined by reference to, the actions of the brain. If the brain acts as a vehicle of or conduit for 'mind', the two cannot be one and the same. To use a metaphor from the Bhagavad Gita, the charioteer needs to be in control of his chariot, but there should be no confusion as to where the chariot ends and where the charioteer begins. Chariot and charioteer function effectively as one, but that does not make them one and the same. Especially with regard to the processes of healing,[4] mind is like the charioteer, that is, effectively in control, whereas brain is merely the chariot. Healing is therefore what comes about when mind and brain, healer and healed, work together in harmony.

Spirituality, Self-discipline and Health

If spirituality is denied, it does not cease to exist, and truth relations do not have to be observed or understood in order for them to exist. Human conditioning means that understanding is always partial.

Science, which usually concerns itself with verifiable facts, provides only partial explanations about the real nature of existence. Spirituality and health go hand in hand, and whether or not the necessary relation is perceived, science is an essential part of this formulation.

Spiritual philosophy can exert a positive influence on how someone conducts his or her life, thereby allowing individuals a high degree of self-control, including accepting a measure of responsibility for their own health. It is possible, therefore, for an individual to help bring about 'inner healing', in so doing making the physical body less prone to illness, especially with regard to illnesses affecting the mind. This holistic, Ayurvedic reasoning (essentially the yoga of health and healing) is one with the philosophy of ancient yoga traditions.

Now is the time to pause and explore some of the ancient aphorisms themselves. In Book II *sloka* 15 of the *Yoga Sutras*, one reads that *Parinama-tapa-samskara-duhkhair guna-vrtti-virodhac ca duhkham eva sarvam vivehinah* (Taimni 1961: 161); or 'Change, anxiety and mental impressions cause sorrow and conflict, even with the wise, on account of the modifications of the mind and the workings of the *gunas*, or characteristic properties of matter' (Worthington 1987: 11).[5] This has modern resonance, when society is changing so fast that people experience levels of anxiety that are not conducive to general wellbeing. Nothing can be done about the external world insofar as 'stopping life' is not an option, but something can be done about *how* individuals respond to external change and to this external environment.

One of the main causes of suffering is described as attachment to the pursuit of pleasure and happiness;[6] another is the extreme avoidance of suffering (Worthington 1987: 10). Suffering is part of human existence, and people often forget that pleasure and pain are two sides of the same coin. Just as success cannot fully be experienced without having known failure, happiness will not come about unless suffering has been experienced. Neither suffering nor the pursuit of happiness is an end in itself, and reacting in the wrong way to things that cannot be changed leads to internal tension, which over time is not good for health.

By the continued practice of the *asanas* (yoga postures), 'one is then no longer assaulted by the pairs of opposites', according to Patanjali (Worthington 1987: 14). Such practice should be effective as a means of promoting healing and coping with the external stresses and strains that characterise modern life. Traditions that go back thousands of years support this claim. While there is much more to *Raja Yoga* than the simple practice of *asana*s, the point about opposites serves as a reminder that wholeness and wellbeing ought to be attainable.

A less well-known text is the *Siva Sutras*, and it is a rich source of information, offering scientific explanations about mind and consciousness (see Worthington 2002). Its subject matter is at the same time spiritual, and while these aphoristic teachings are of unknown origin, they are strongly identified with Mount Kailash, which is high up in the Himalayas. They are very condensed and it needs sustained effort in order to be able to try and fathom their meaning. Book I, about the realisation of the Self, describes how *Vitarka atma-jnanam* or 'Self-knowledge arises from continuous reflection on the *atma*, or spirit of consciousness' (ibid.: 29). This captures the idea of the need for sustained effort in order to attain the fruits of inner self-discipline.

Self-discipline may seem alien to people living in a fast-moving, modern world, but because of the speed of change it becomes more, not less, important to be able to practice inner discipline. Social change, such as that taking place in the early 21st century, can in this way be seen as instructive, rather than damaging or harmful. Checks and balances serve to mitigate the extremes of happiness and sorrow, and so, in some ways, readjustments taking place within the social order can lead people to pause a while, creating time to examine the inner self. If healing brings together healer and the healed, the path of self-knowledge and self-discipline ought to be followed by anyone interested in restoring connections between what is perceived as real, and what simply *is*. This ideal may seem too remote for many people to adopt in ordinary everyday life; nonetheless, it can be seen how science and spirituality work together in harmony, and how each is in many ways integral to the other, especially with regard to the different modes of healing.

The *Siva Sutra*s give an account of four discrete states of consciousness: normal waking consciousness, ordinary sleep, dreamless sleep, and a fourth state, which transcends the other three, known as *turiya* or supreme consciousness. *Sutra* 3.21 reads: *Magnah svacittena praviset*, which translates as: 'The fourth state entered into by immersion in the inner consciousness, is marked by clarity of understanding' (Worthington 2002: 89). This state is said to transcend the other three (normal) states of consciousness. While knowledge of this state can really only come about by experiencing it, the mere fact that there is such a state indicates that there is an alternative explanation to the visible, material universe.

The real secrets of healing may be found locked within this fourth state. Granted, to know that this state exists is not the same as to experience it; nonetheless, it opens up the possibility in such a way that connections can be said to exist between the seen and unseen, and between the physical and non-physical worlds. These are beyond normal perceptions, which might help to explain what is otherwise a hidden mystery. All in all, there is infinite depth to be found within Himalayan thought, not least when it comes to considerations about the science of healing and the different states of consciousness.

Notes

1. Traditionally, there are seven schools of yoga, of which raja is one and hatha is another, the others being mantra, kundalini, laya, karma, and bhakti yoga.
2. See Book IV, *Kaivalya-pada*, or The Book of Liberation of Yoga Sutras (Taimni 1961: 377–446; Worthington 1987: 38–47).
3. In Book II, *The Practice of Yoga,* or *Sadhana-pada*, *sloka*s 4 and 5 read: *Avidya ksetram uttaresam prsaupta-tanu-vicchinnodaranam*, and *Anityasuci-duhkhanamasu nitya-suci-sukhatmakhyatir avidya* (Taimni 1961: 138–40), which translate as 'Ignorance is the source of the other kleshas (causes of sorrow or suffering), whether they are in a dormant, attenuated or active state', and '*Avidya* is mistaking the non-eternal, the impure, the sorrow-ful and the non-spirit for their opposites', respectively (Worthington 1987: 10).
4. In Book I of the Gita, Arjuna and Krishna ride into battle on a chariot. Arjuna is the warrior and Krishna his charioteer. Together they achieve victory: Arjuna making great effort and Krishna exhibiting great skill in controlling the chariot, whilst giving advice and instruction to Arjuna. The chariot is merely the necessary vehicle that contributed to, but did not cause, success in their great endeavour. Similarly, the mind is the causal agent, not the brain. Only when the brain malfunctions does it become an agent of causation, in a way that is not dissimilar to a wheel falling off the chariot and leading to disaster.
5. This, and all further references to the *Yoga Sutras*, are from Worthington (1987, 2002), unless specified.
6. Mistaking the real for the unreal is one of the chief causes of sorrow, according to Patanjali (see YS II.3 in Worthington 1987: 10).

References

Taimni, I. K. 1961. *The Science of Yoga.* Chicago: Theosophical Publishing House.

Worthington, R. 1987. *A Student's Companion to Patanjali.* London: Theosophical Publishing House.

———. 2002. *The Hidden Self: A Study of the Siva Sutras.* Philadelphia: Himalayan Institute Press.

Five

The Culture and Philosophy of Bio-medicine in India

Critical Sociological Reflections

Suhita Chopra Chatterjee

Bio-medicine is a distinctly Western system of healing. But it has been taken up, researched and practised in a variety of cultural contexts, which then influences its practice. Among other elements, the politico-economic context and ideas about health and illness especially shape these practices. Researchers have therefore argued that rather than as a single entity, bio-medicine may be viewed as a plurality of bio-medicines that are socially and culturally situated (Good 1995: 462). Further, M. J. Good and B. J. Good write:

> The globalization of biomedical cultures and the political economies of medicine has had a profound influence on local and cosmopolitan cultures of clinical medicine world-wide. Nevertheless, although bio-medicine is fostered through an international political economy of biotechnology and by an international community of medical educators and bioscientists, it still is taught, practiced, organized, and consumed in local contexts (2000: 243).

Drawing insight from Good and Good's understanding, we may try to analyse 'Bio-medicine in India'. This chapter examines the culture and philosophy of bio-medicine in India in light of the current understanding of its features in the West. Admittedly, examining all aspects of bio-medicine (organisational structure, financing, governance, policy, medical education, and research) is a formidable task. This chapter is therefore more narrowly, and less ambitiously, structured around a central concern — to examine whether bio-medicine has been able to adapt itself to the Indian socio-cultural reality. In pursuing this concern, the chapter tries to show that the enabling structural factors for the emergence of bio-medicine as a science are not uniformly present in India. As a result, the culture that it has engendered does not do full justice to India's unique concern for an equitable health sector. Culturally, too, it remains disembedded from and alien to Indian society.

The Culture and Philosophy of Bio-medicine in the West

Perhaps the best exposition of this is to be found in A. Kleinman's article, titled, 'What is specific to Bio-medicine?' He highlights many features to show the fragmented and reductionist orientation of bio-medicine, and makes special mention of its 'extreme insistence on materialism as the grounds of knowledge' and 'discomfort with dialectical modes of thought'. He writes, 'single causal chains must be used to specify pathogenesis in a language of structural flaws and mechanisms as the rationale for therapeutic efficacy' (1995: 29). The insistence on materialism as the grounds of knowledge has resulted in a particular way of looking at the body, with a special emphasis on 'seeing'. The primacy of materialistic entities makes no room for a patient's suffering in the therapeutic vision. According to Kleinman:

> The patient's and family's complaints are regarded as *subjective* self-reports, biased accounts of a too-personal somewhere. The physician's task, wherever possible is to replace these biased observations with *objective* data: the only valid sign of pathological processes, because they are based on verified and verifiable measurements (1995: 32).

Further, Kleinman observes that bio-medicine, 'because of its long development under the powerful regimen of industrial capitalism', is also 'the most institutionalized of the forms of medicine' (ibid.: 37). Bio-medicine is both bureaucracy and profession. Rules and regulations control practice, and the doctor is the provider of a product that is advertised, marketed and sold. The technical rationality of the institution, its priorities and norms govern its practice: 'The very imagery of care constructs an industrial logic to its delivery and evaluation, reducing the moral space of the carrier of illness and of the work of doctoring to a minimum' (ibid.: 37–38). Professionalisation is equally important for bio-medicine. If 'bureaucratization routinizes efficiency', 'professionalization routinizes the "quality" of care' (ibid.: 38).

The most powerful and controversial attribute of bio-medicine is its ability to construct various forms of human suffering as health problems. Its constructions then influence different sectors of experience. In other words, 'it is a leading institution of industrialized society's management of social realty' (Kleinman 1995: 38). In the construction of health and illness, it leaves no room for alternative paradigms of healing.

Over the years, this very succinct characterisation of bio-medicine has emerged as a major feature of its development in the West. Bio-medicine has become more of a science than an art of healing. And it is Big Science, entrenched in the capitalist ethos and marked by the emergence of excessively high-technology tertiary-care institutions as a prominent feature of healthcare delivery.

Although not within the purview of this chapter, it may be recalled briefly that the infusion of science and the scientific method in bio-medicine is of fairly recent origin, and coincides with developments in the larger field of Western science. E. Shorter, in trying to understand the larger chronicle of changes in the history of the doctor–patient relationship, holds that three crucial events in the 19th century infused the scientific method in the practice of medicine. These are: advances in clinical examination, pathological anatomy, and microbiology (Shorter 1993). But it was in the beginning of 1935 that the advent of wonder drugs like Protonsil or benzenesulphonamide and penicillin prompted research into bio-chemical and pharmacological mechanisms. The post-modern period thus began in the years after World War II, and the dominant approach to medical education in the 1950s was to treat medical students as mini-scientists rather than physicians to be. The tilt towards science in the medical curriculum was rationalised on the grounds that the physician must understand the scientific mechanisms underlying the drugs prescribed. The great Internist of Columbia University, Robert Loeb (1895–1973), pronounced the last rites in 1953 of social sciences and training in home-care programmes, aspiring only for standards of the highest possible scientific level.

From 1960 onwards, other developments in technology further scienticised medicine. Computers started making an advent in medicine, and by the 1990s, they became ubiquitous in monitoring physiological functions, analysing electrical signals from machines, managing systems, and in the precise control of delicate interventions, such as drug infusion or therapy. But it soon became evident that like other diagnostic technologies preceding its use, computers depend upon the user's self-image, human relationships and social standing. They are not only extensions of the user's physical and intellectual selves, but also of their personalities (Reiser 1993). However, these developments in technology did bring in a lot of changes in consultation techniques. Attention to laboratory data and diagnostic imaging replaced painstaking interest in detailed history-taking, and the whole approach to the patient as a person. In other words, a high technology-oriented science of medicine emerged.

Bio-medicine's alliance with science is perhaps one of the reasons for its dominance in the West. It was in accord with the larger aims and goals of science and knowledge production in science. The history of medicine in the West shows that it was also in accord with the political culture in which the continuing negotiations between the institution of medicine and the state took place to support each other's overt and covert goals (Fox 1993). In general, the state supported many of the goals — providing medical services for the poor, spreading equitably the cost of illness, governing and subsidising hospital services, and organising medical education, to name a few. In many Western societies, healthcare policies of the state were grounded in the liberal political tradition. These were focused on norms of personal wellbeing and individual freedom, and were concerned with protecting as well as assuring rights and its underlying distributive-justice paradigm. This framework guided policy debates regarding universal health insurance, welfare reforms for the vulnerable, issues about the rising costs of medical care, and the growing dominance of market-oriented care. Civil rights and women's rights movements also developed wings, especially directed towards increasing access to healthcare, changing the quality of healthcare, and reforming the caring professions (Epstein 2008).

The centrality of technology in bio-medicine was also congruent with the liberal democratic order. The state tried to present itself as neutral to competing group interests. Bio-medicine, like other fields of science, could accomplish this agenda of political neutrality through technical rationality, impersonality, and the objective presentation of facts.

Culturally, bio-medicine was congruent with the Western view of human beings. Even the focus on the body was in accord with the Western emphasis on the individual. As Benoist and Cathebras pointed out, 'One of the functions of the body becomes that of marking the frontiers of the individual' (1993: 858). The separation of the mind and body offered a subtle articulation of the person's alienation from the body in Western society — a feature found in every sphere of economic and political life as well.

Interestingly, bio-medicine's narrow, fragmented and scientific perspective evoked considerable criticism from various quarters. The rising costs of treatment, diagnostic errors, escalations in iatrogenic[1] diseases, and bio-medicine's inability to deal effectively with diseases like AIDS and cancer drew considerable critique from the social sciences (see Illich 1976; Lupton 2003; Turner 1992). Politico-economic theorists were extremely sceptical of developments in medicine. Considering health as not only a bio-medical reality but also a social, economic and political issue, they cautioned against the healthcare system under capitalism. According to them, greater spending on health does not necessarily lead to a better status of health. Neither does universal access to health care lead to universal good health. Little of any long-term gains in health are due to clinical medicine. In fact, they argued that most tests and procedures are unnecessary. In other words, the credibility of the medical profession was seriously challenged. The social constructionists did not call into question illness, disease states, or bodily experiences, but emphasised that these states should be known and examined using cultural and social understanding. The field of cultural studies, too, emphasised people's understanding of the world, including their beliefs about medicine and disease, and the need to culturally embed bio-medicine.

Perhaps the most vocal criticism came from the post-modernists, who heralded a series of changes in people's understanding of science and scientific epistemology. According to them, a concern with objectivism does not make subjective ideas redundant. There has to be an epistemologically legitimate space for subjective aspects of illness — the patient's desires, thinking, behaviour, fear, feeling, and emotion, and also the social contexts that govern each of these emotions. Post-modernists questioned the excessive 'medicalisation' and 'technologisation' of medicine. Within the epistemological boundary of post-modern medicine, they created a space for religion and spiritual knowledge. In general, they contributed to a growing disenchantment with science.

The growing dissent from various quarters led the World Health Organization (WHO) to adopt a more expansive definition of health as a state of complete physical, mental and social wellbeing, and not merely the absence of disease or infirmity. A bio-psycho-social model of health, rather than a bio-medical model, began to be appreciated

(Engel 1977). Health promotion (which emphasises broader structural and strategic interventions involving different sectors) rather than health care gained prominence. There was a flight towards demedicalisation and a return to alternative medicines as well.[2] The concept of palliative care (which integrates psychological and spiritual dimensions of care) implicitly signalled the limits of medicine, and its inability to sustain high-cost technological interventions in end-of-life care. In general, there was pressure on the state to revise the social contract with medical institutions in order to redistribute resources — away from clinical medicine and bio-medical research, towards learning more about the social determinants of health and devising policies and practices based on such knowledge.

Bio-medicine in India: The Local Culture of Bio-medicine and its Cultural Manifestations

When we now turn to bio-medicine in India, we find that its organisation of knowledge and practice is based on the Western scientific tradition. Beginning as an art form, it has, over the years, turned into a science, and in the process imbibed the features which Kleinman has so succinctly identified. The underlying philosophy of the medical model has been adopted, with its emphasis on pathologies and clinical intervention. Bio-medicine has evolved into being high technology-oriented and science-centred, as seen in super-specialty hospitals, which has lent itself to excessive bureaucratisation and professionalisation. But while in many advanced countries of the West the politico-economic culture is geared to sustain the high level of technical rationality required for the proper functioning of the medical system, in India, its development is marred by the sheer lack of pre-requisites for such transformation. An effective and sustainable medical system needs to be backed by good governance, a sound health policy (particularly in matters related to finance) involving a good deal of civic groundwork — building an audience, creating a broad-based support system, creating awareness and linkages between health and other social sectors,[3] and an adequate health information system capable of efficient data generation and tracking systems integrated with allied health sciences. So far, post-independence, the politico-economic culture in India has not proved itself capable of sustaining a scientific-technocratic medical culture throughout India. The result is that India sees the best and the worst in the field of bio-medical development.[4]

The state's role in financing bio-medicine has been very poor. Bio-medicine — the Big Science — requires big money. But public spending on health in India, as a percentage of GDP, is less than in countries like Sri Lanka and Sierra Leone. Currently, India spends close to 3 per cent of its GDP on education and less than 1 per cent of its GDP on health (for details, see Wada Na Todo Abhiyan 2013), and this is largely limited to family planning, immunisation, selected disease surveillance, medical education, and research. To make matters worse, there is a high degree of privatisation of health care. According to the World Bank, India has one of the highest levels of private financing; 84 per cent of health care is out-of-pocket expenses. Naturally, the system is set up to favour those who can pay. The ambitious goal of providing universal health care for all has so far not been achieved.

State policies with respect to economic development have been unable to prioritise health within the overall development. The reductionist bio-medical approach to health has further accentuated the problem. A slow and modest pace of poverty reduction, despite the robust economic growth in India in the last Five-Year Plan,[5] worsening regional imbalances with inter-state inequalities, poor employment growth, and unfavourable working conditions have impacted the health of the population, solutions to which cannot be provided by only a fragmented approach to disease (see Radhakrishna 2008).

Operating within the context of marked regional economic imbalances and inter-state inequalities in per capita State Domestic Product (SDP), bio-medicine, with its high-cost technological orientation, has reinforced and perpetuated existing social inequalities and divides between the privileged and the underprivileged. Thus, health status inequities have worsened in backward states like Bihar, Orissa and Uttar Pradesh. For example, in Gaya district in Bihar, only 5 per cent of children were fully immunised, whereas in Tumkur district, Karnataka, in southern India, the level of child immunisation has reached more than 90 per cent. Orissa has an MMR of 358 per 1,00,000 live births, whereas Kerala, with the highest literacy rate, has an MMR of 110 per 1,00,000 live births. Rural–urban differences in healthcare provision have also become stark and glaring. There are 585 rural hospitals compared to 985 urban hospitals in the country. Of the 6,39,729 doctors registered in India, only 67,576 are in the public sector. The ratio of hospital beds to population in rural areas is almost 15 times lower than that for urban areas (Wada Na Todo Abhiyan 2007).

One of the reasons for such inequities is the fact that bio-medicine, like all other scientific enterprises, can only select identifiable geographical locations, which constitute privileged sites, for its practice and research. According to scholars, 'place' matters a great deal for the practices and accomplishments of science. Globalised science is at the same time *emplaced* science; it takes place at identifiable geographic locations and amidst special architectural and material circumstances that acquire a distinctive cultural meaning (Henke and Gieryn 2008).

In terms of governance, too, the situation is rather grim. While standardisation activities were central in the transformation of healing practices into scientific-technological medicine in the West, in India, the attempts to standardise clinical practice guidelines through payment patterns, clinical decision-making, and codes of conduct have been unsatisfactory.

State regulatory mechanisms for clinical trials and drug manufacturing have evoked considerable concern because of their poor results in reducing the variability of practices and products that create inefficiencies. Moreover, unlike in the West, health reform has not emerged as the cornerstone of the civil rights movement in India. Wherever they exist, they do not seem to have adopted a strong oppositional position against bio-medicine.[6]

Is Bio-medicine Culturally Disembedded?

The absence of enabling factors for an efficient culture of bio-medicine may be shown ad infinitum. However, the intention is not to dwell on these, but to demonstrate that it is this science-based culture of medicine (inappropriately developed and incongruent with the local context) that has impeded a proper understanding of health and illness in India. Given the disease-oriented perspective, bio-medicine has failed to generate alternative conceptualisations which can look at health in the local socio-economic context. This is evident from the fact that even the health status and health infrastructure indicators used in India have been derived and developed in the West. They not only fail to question the attending bias and value-judgements inherent in Western models of health, but also show poor sensitivity to the people's own way of defining health within their unique social-cultural norms. For instance, maternal health is gauged by 'percent of births delivered in the hospitals'. One could legitimately ask: Whose value judgement is imbibed in such an indicator, which puts a premium on hospital vis-à-vis home births? One is reminded here of development indicators that were extensively used in the 1960s and 1970s, till scholars asked the question, 'for whom and why', and suggested 'putting people first' (Cernea 1985).

Returning to the birth indicators, do they convey local choices and people's values? Do they reflect the current value shift worldwide in favour of the new natural birthing movement which gives women more control over their bodies? Do they capture the essence of social science literature on these issues, and the government's own commitment to training *dais* (local women who traditionally helped to deliver babies in pre-modern India) in a serious effort to provide for the people's preference for a non-medicalised perspective on birthing? Do they put people first, enabling them to live their own lives as they wish? Are the authorities confident that services are safe and of high quality, and that they promote individual needs for independence, wellbeing and dignity? Finally, does health care for woman include not merely pregnancy and childbirth, but the entire spectrum of her life?

The dominant emphasis on the medical model has not only done poor justice to cultural factors, but has also, so far, failed to understand disease in the broader social context in which the pursuit of health and responses to this are shaped. Thus, diseases like tuberculosis, malaria and, more recently, AIDS, have been considered without due cognisance of the social context of poverty and malnutrition. The emphasis in AIDS prevention has been more on the pathogen which causes the disease, rather than on the complex social issues which lead to the suppression of immunity and predispose people to risky sexual behaviour. Similarly, the approach towards maternal death often only captures the immediate biological and medical causes, overlooking the personal, familial, socio-cultural, and environmental factors behind crucial delays leading to death.

Many bio-medical interventions for public health have also failed to yield successful results due to the superimposition of Western and alien modes of thinking on the local populace, without amalgamating lay explanations with medical discourses. In a study on thalassaemia, it was found that even if health services were provided, some ethnic groups may not avail of the full range of available medical interventions because of their moralistic association of thalassaemia with sexually improper marriage liaisons (Roy 2007). Given the multi-cultural composition of Indian society, it seems imperative to generate systematic data in access research with a view to merging social science research information with health policy and medical concerns.

That bio-medicine in India has failed to weave its theory and practice with Indian cultural values is also evident in the design of IEC programmes, which have often generated hostility among the target populations. For instance, the educational brochures for AIDS prevention designed by international agencies have evoked strong resistance from various hill communities because of the supposedly offensive symbolisms and meanings conveyed by the pictorial representations of the body and sexuality. In some cases, the images of playful sexuality associated with condoms have impeded their success as a prophylactic device, since they come in the way of reproductive sex.

Perhaps the most blatant neglect has been in matters of medical prescription, which has rarely done justice to people's ways of understanding medicine and its impact on the body. A patient's compliance to medical prescriptions and methods of ingesting medicines shows deep cultural beliefs. For instance, medicines, particularly antibiotics, in India continue to be imbued with the property of 'heat', even among the well-educated, leading to their indiscriminate withdrawal. Or, in contravention of popular medical opinion, they are ingested with milk due to the latter's inherent healing properties, thereby reducing their therapeutic efficacy. Communicating with patients with distinctly different health beliefs requires sensitivity and training, and a highly individualised approach. The narrative structures used by patients in a therapeutic encounter in India are different and require sensitive de-coding. Also, it seems that the therapeutic relationship of the impersonal consumer type does not hold good in India where, till recently, paternalistic relationships were important.

An equally disembedded approach is reflected in technology deployment. The assessment of the need for technology — type and level of technology use, cultural alternatives to technology deployment, ethical issues about specific technological interventions, particularly invasive technologies, their cost and use-effectiveness in India — has not been systematically researched. Technology deployment decisions related to end-of-life care have been insensitive to Indian conceptions of life, death and body, and the financial implications on families.[7] Debates about technology use need special consideration in the context of women's health and illness. Assisted conception technologies, excessive use of prenatal screening technologies,[8] and the technical and changing nature of childbirth in obstetrical procedures all need to be re-evaluated for their role in Indian culture. There is also a need to review medical technology in the diagnosis of asymptomatic diseases. In other words, cultural sensitivity requires developing a distinctly Indian code of medical ethics on technology use.

Finally, like bio-medicine in the West, bio-medicine in India too has a trained insensitivity to medical pluralism. The growing trend towards science-based medicine has led to the conceptual gulf between bio-medicine and indigenous medicine growing increasingly wide. The growing confidence in the power of Western science has challenged the basis of indigenous medicine and strengthened the monopolistic domination of science-based medicine. At best, bio-medicine has sought the integration of alternative medicines with its own theory and philosophy, rather than integrate itself with the alternative healing systems in India. As a result, the government-funded parallel infrastructure of traditional health facilities and trained personnel are not utilised for either public health programmes or primary healthcare (Misra et al. 2003).

Conclusion

This chapter shows that the organisation of bio-medical knowledge and practice in India is based on Western scientific traditions. It reflects the epistemological and ontological commitments of the scientific paradigm. However, the broader politico-economic and organisational structure, which sustains any efficient use of technology, and the tilt towards science in medicine is lacking in India. There is also a lack of cultural congruence between bio-medicine and local moral experiences and beliefs about health and illness.

However, it is not merely the absence of enabling structures (good governance, resource allocation, human resources, physical access, removal of social barriers, etc.) and cultural incongruence that consolidates this disparity between bio-medicine and the socio-cultural context in which it is practised. There is an inevitability in bio-medicine's own bureaucratic, highly consumerist, fragmented, and purely disease-oriented approach to health, which results in the sort of inefficiencies that the health sector witnesses in India. It prompts one to ask: In developing countries like India, is it not time for bio-medicine to re-evaluate its role? Given the existing scenario of socio-eco-political underdevelopment in large parts of the country, should it not profess to be less of a science and more of an art, more humane and less professional, more integrated than specialised, more oriented to health than disease, more equitable than competitive, more community-oriented rather than market-driven? And, most important of all, given the evidence of its own failure in improving the health of the nation, should bio-medicine not try to integrate itself with alternative medicine in India, rather than seeking their integration with its own philosophy and practice?

In questioning the level and desirability of the scientific and technocratic medical culture in India, in raising the question of whether medicine is best appreciated as an art or a science, we need to assure ourselves that this is not ethno-solipsism. Many of the issues raised in this chapter have formed the cornerstone of an ongoing criticism of bio-medicine in the West. In fact, many corrections have already been made in the dominant model of health and illness in Western countries. Perhaps what we need is greater sensitivity and awareness of these paradigmatic shifts in bio-medicine in order to redefine its culture and practice to suit Indian reality.

Notes

1. 'Relating to illness caused by medical examination or treatment' (Oxford Dictionaries Online) http://oxforddictionaries.com.
2. In most Western countries, there has been a steady growth in the use of Complementary and Alternative Medicines (CAM). Americans spend as much on CAM as on hospitalisation. According to a recent survey, 28 per cent of adults in England had used one of eight types of complementary medicine in the past one year (Marks et al. 2005). Unfortunately, in some parts of the world, despite their popularity, CAM are under increasing pressure from health professionals to meet positivist scientific standards of safety and efficiency (Kelner et al. 2003: 915–30).
3. The need for more integral approaches and inter-sectoral synergies in the health sector has become sufficiently clear in the case of the Millennium Development Goals. For instance, the World Bank has noted that physical infrastructure, transport and roads are complementary to health services. A 10-year study in Rajasthan found that better roads and transport helped women reach referral facilities more easily. But many died anyway because there were no corresponding improvements to sustain it (Wagstaf and Claeson 2004).
4. The health sector provides a picture of contrasts. On the one hand, even primary health centres in many parts of India are understaffed and

ill-equipped, and on the other, India has seen enormous growth in medical tourism due to its low-cost advantage and new high-quality healthcare services. Approximately 1,50,000 patients arrived in 2004 from across the globe for medical treatment, from countries like the US, UK, the Middle East, Africa, and SAARC countries. The medical tourism market in India, estimated at US$ 333 million in 2004, grew by about 25 per cent, and was predicted to become a US$ 2 billion-a-year business opportunity by 2012 (Equity Bulls 2006).

5. Despite sustained high GDP growth in India, estimates of global poverty by World Bank in 2008 suggest that India has more people living below US$ 2 than even sub-Saharan Africa. India has 456 million people, or around 42 per cent of its population living below the new international poverty line of $1.25 a day. The number of Indian poor constitutes 33 per cent of the global poor, pegged at 1.4 billion people (Oneworld South Asia 2008). India-Urban Poverty Report 2009 shows that there are over 80 million poor people living in the cities and towns of India (Ministry of Housing and Urban Poverty Alleviation, Government of India 2009).
6. A notable exception in recent times is Swami Ramdev's attempt to popularise Pranayama Yoga and Ayurveda. The movement questions not only the dominance of Western medicine, but also the entire philosophical foundation that underpins the modern worldview that medical science holds the key to a disease-free society. Despite this opposition, however, it uses Western science's method of legitimation — the empirico-rational method — for presenting the therapeutic outcomes to the masses.
7. The increasing resort to ICUs and the use of expensive technologies in it is causing a dilemma in Indian society. It is not uncommon for those working in ICUs to be asked by anxious relatives, 'how long will this patient need to stay in ICU? We are running out of funds' (Pandya 2005: 79–96).
8. In India, not much is known about the meanings of prenatal technologies. In contradiction to the stated objectives of the MTP Act 1971, sex selection has emerged as a primary reason for their deployment, indicating a major transmutation of meanings in technologies. It is estimated that in the late 1990s, more than 100,000 sex-selective abortions of female foetuses were being performed annually in India, leading to a skewed sex ratio of 107–21 males per 100 females in 16 of India's 26 states in 1998–99 (Arnold et al. 2002). One also needs to assess whether the prevailing cultural assumption in the West, namely that foreknowledge is essentially good, is relevant in India as well. While prenatal diagnosis in the West helps to prepare parents and doctors for the birth of a baby with a structural or genetic problem, in a developing country with poor postnatal facilities, the disconnect between testing and the right to treatment/termination may constitute a 'Tyranny of diagnosis'.

References

Arnold, F., Sunita Kishor and T. K. Roy. 2002. 'Sex-Selective Abortions in India', *Population and Development Review*, 28 (4): 759–85.

Benoist, J. and P. Cathebras. 1993. 'The Body: From an Immateriality to Another', *Social Science and Medicine*, 36: 857–65.

Cernea, Michael M. (ed.). 1985. *Putting People First: Sociological Variables in Rural Development*. New York: Oxford University Press.

Engel, G. L. 1977. 'The Need for a New Medical Model: A Challenge for Bio-medicine', *Science*, 196: 129–36.

Epstein, S. 2008. 'Patient Groups and Health Movements', in E. J. Hackett and Society for the Study of Social Sciences (eds), *The Handbook of Science and Technology Studies*, pp. 499–539. Cambridge: MIT Press.

Equity Bulls. 2006. 'Ministry of Tourism Promotes Medical Tourism in India', *Equity Bulls*, http://www.equitybulls.com/admin/news2006/news_det.asp?id=17762 (accessed 3 April 2013).

Fox, Daniel M. 1993. 'Medical Institutions and the State', in A. F. Bynum and Roy Porter (eds), *The Companion Encyclopedia of the History of Medicine*, pp. 1204–30. London: Routledge.

Good, M. J. 1995. 'Cultural Studies of Bio-medicine: An Agenda for Research', *Social Science and Medicine*, 41: 461–63.

Good, M. J. and B. J. Good. 2000. 'Clinical Narratives and the Study of Contemporary Doctor-Patient Relationships', in Albrecht Gary et al. (eds), *Handbook of Social Studies in Health and Medicine*, pp. 243–58. London: Sage Publications.

Henke, Christopher R. and F. Thomas Gieryn. 2008. 'Sites of Scientific Medicine: The Enduring Importance of Place', in E. J. Hackett and Society for the Study of Social Sciences (eds), *The Handbook of Science and Technology Studies*, pp. 353–76. Cambridge: MIT Press.

Illich, I. 1976. *Limits to Medicine*. London: Calder and Boyars.

Kelner, M., B. Wellman, H. Boon, and S. Welsh. 2003. 'Responses of Established Healthcare to the Professionalization of Complementary and Alternative Medicine in Ontario', *Social Science and Medicine*, 59 (5): 915–30.

Kleinman, A. 1995. *Writing at the Margin: Discourse between Anthropology and Medicine*. Berkeley: University of Berkeley Press.

Lupton, D. 2003. *Medicine as Culture*. London: Sage Publications.

Marks, David F., Michael Murray, Brian Evans, Emee Vida Estacio (eds). 2005. *Health Psychology: Theory Research and Practice*. London: Sage Publications.

Ministry of Housing and Urban Poverty Alleviation, Government of India. 2009. 'India: Urban Poverty Report 2009: Factsheet', *India | United Nations Development Programme*, http://www.in.undp.org/content/dam/india/docs/india_urban_poverty_report_2009.pdf (accessed 3 April 2013).

Misra, Rajiv, Rachel Chatterjee and Sujatha Rao (eds). 2003. *India Health Report*. New Delhi: Oxford University Press.

Oneworld South Asia. 2008. 'Fresh figures suggest poverty in India still staggering', *Oneworld South Asia*, http://southasia.oneworld.net/news/world-bank-figures-suggest-poverty-in-india-still-staggering#.UVwUzJNTB9Q (accessed 3 April 2013).

Pandya, Sunil K. 2005. 'End of Life Decision-Making in India', in R. H. Blank and Janna C. Merrick (eds), *End of Life Decision-making: A Cross National Study*. Cambridge: MIT Press.

Radhakrishna, R. and Indira Gandhi Institute of Development Research (eds). 2008. *India Development Report*. New York: Oxford University Press.

Reiser, Stanley Joel. 1993. 'The Science of Diagnosis', in A. F. Bynum and Roy Porter (eds), *The Companion Encyclopedia of the History of Medicine*. London: Routledge.

Roy, Tanuka. 2007. 'Illness Experiences: A Sociological Study of Adolescent Thalassaemics and Their Parent Caregivers', Ph.D. dissertation, IIT Kharagpur.

Shorter, E. 1993. 'The History of the Doctor-Patient Relationship', in A. F. Bynum and Roy Porter (eds), *The Companion Encyclopedia of the History of Medicine*. London: Routledge.

Sudarshan, H. 2008. 'Governance in Health Services', in K. V. Ramani, D. Mavalankar and D. Govil (eds), *Strategic Issues and Challenges in Health Management*. New Delhi: Sage Publications.

Turner, B. 1992. *Regulating Bodies: Essays in Medical Sociology*. London: Routledge.

Wada Na Todo Abhiyan. 2007. 'Ensuring Universal Access to Health and Education in India: Executive Summary', *Wada Na Todo Abhiyan*, http://www.wadanatodo.net/camapaignreports/healtheducation.asp (accessed 3 April 2013).

Wagstaf, A. and Mariam Claeson. 2004. *The Millennium Development Goals for Health: Rising to the Challenges*. Washington DC: World Bank.

Six

Spirituality, Mental Health and Perfectionism

Nilanjana Sanyal

Attainment of psychological wellbeing is the main pursuit of an education that enhances the quality of one's life. This is all the more apparent when addressing issues of ill-health in psychological clinics. Experience in clinical psychology prompts the understanding that true 'meaning-setting' in life, or spiritual attainment, should be the goal of life's journey. But the growing trend of materialistic pursuits is laying stress on just the opposite — being rigid, moralistic, inflexible, in order to truly be a 'perfectionist'. This dilemma needs theoretical probing.

Psychological wealth is the experience of wellbeing and a high quality of life. It is more than simple fleeting joy and more than an absence of depression and anxiety. Psychological health is the perception that our life is excellent — that there are ways in life to feel rewarded, engaged and meaningful, while enjoying life's bounties. It also includes a sense of satisfaction, of engagement in interesting activities, the pursuit of important goals, the experience of positive emotional feelings, and a sense of spirituality that connects people to things larger than themselves. In addition to the internal aspects of the concept of psychological health, there are universal benchmarks of a fulfilled and rewarding life, such as health and positive social relationships. These constitute the external facets of psychological health (Diener and Biswas-Diener 2008). Hence, in the framework of psychological health and wealth, the essential components seem to be:

- Physical and mental health.
- Engaging activities and work.
- Material sufficiency to take care of basic needs.
- Positive attitudes and emotions.
- Values and life-goals to achieve.

- Loving social relationships.
- Satisfaction with life, and happiness.
- Spirituality and meaning in life.

Attaining this state of psychological wealth is not an easy task. The whole process needs a movement through sequential developmental phases. In fact, humans have a long period of development — from infancy through puberty — during which we depend strongly upon others. Adults with their experiences and dictums stand as points of reference for the young child who follows the examples set before her/him, initially only to gain approval and be happy. Relationships matter to our emotional wellbeing and psychological health because the fabric of our close relationships directly influences us in a variety of ways. We blossom from children into adults only through the encouragement, support and mentorship of parents, teachers, guides, and other significant associates in our lives. The concept of adherence to dictated norms, of being disciplined, organised, regimented, and therefore 'perfect', is embedded here. This is the story of early mental development. The problem with such adherence in order to gain approval and become 'perfect' in the eyes of the world is that it may generate narrowness of vision and mission, lack of a drive for personal experience, ignorance of one's creative potential, and resistance towards the true enjoyment of life.

Conceptual Framework of Mental Health as the Baseline of Psychological Wellbeing

The basic tenets of mental health indicate that adaptation is the psychological mechanism that governs one's emotional baseline. Adjusting to new circumstances allows one to learn new skills, tolerate change, and seek improvement. Adaptation acts as a buffer against trauma in life and prevents one from permanently succumbing to negativity. This resilience is the first indicator of mental health. Thus, mental health is a term used to describe either a level of cognitive or emotional wellbeing, and may include an individual's ability to enjoy life and procure a balance between life activities and efforts to achieve psychological resilience.

The World Health Organization defines mental health as 'a state of wellbeing in which the individual realizes his/her own abilities, can cope with the normal stresses of life, can work productively and fruitfully and is able to make a contribution to his or her community' (2010). Hence, mental wellness is generally viewed as a positive attribute, such that a person can reach enhanced levels of mental health at any turning point in life, which may come about through self-realisation or through therapeutic intervention (Wong 2000). The high-point of mental health is 'emotional well-being', the capacity to live a full and creative life and the flexibility to deal with life's inevitable challenges (Witmer and Sweeny 1992). A holistic model of mental health generally includes content from anthropological, educational, psychological, religious, and sociological perspectives, as well as theoretical notions from personality studies, clinical observations, and elements of developmental psychology. Mental health brings to the surface, at the level of behaviour, an individual's capacity:

- To learn new skills and concepts.
- The ability to feel, express, and manage a range of positive and negative emotions.
- The ability to cope with and manage change and uncertainty (Weare 2000: 12).

The following behavioural features are expected to be present in a mentally healthy person:

- Should possess a sense of contentment and wellbeing.
- Keeps up high spirits and has resilience.
- Participates in life experiences to the full extent.
- The feeling of self-realisation is a must in such a person.
- The self must be flexible in order to deal with the different ordeals of life.
- The ability to strike a balance in the different aspects of life. One needs to be social at times, in solitude at other times, to realise the different facets of life.
- An inclination towards development of health, spirit, body, mind, and soul. A sense of well-roundedness and creativity is imperative.
- Good self-esteem and adequate self-confidence (Keyes 2002).

Taken together, these characteristics point to the importance of having individualised goals, while maintaining a concern for others in our quest for the realisation of the true purpose of life. These are essential in order to have a successful life, especially since we are all subjects of a highly materialistic culture. Ego-adaptation and adjustment is a must in life. The desire for material success is an obvious aspect, but to have real mental health, a disciplined mind must be open to the vast realms of realisation beyond the pale of a materialistic life; it must be open to the serenity and calm that accompanies a transcendental orientation. Mental health and spirituality are thus found to be inseparable.

Spirituality: The Crystal Ball in Life-realisation

Our society is dedicated almost entirely to the celebration of the ego, with all its magniloquent fantasies about success and power. It celebrates those very forces of greed and ignorance that are destroying the beauty of this planet. It will not be an overstatement to say that the entire society is personal-goal oriented, and negates every idea of sacredness and eternal meaning. The net outcome of this is our bewildered mental orientation, a sense of being trapped in a nightmare of our own materialistic creation (Rinpoche 2008). The need for a spiritualistic frame of mind as the carrier of health is very much felt here.

An important aspect of spirituality is the set of positive emotions that connects us to a world larger than ourselves. A deep sense of spirituality based on all-encompassing positive emotions such as love, awe, compassion, and transcendence seems to be necessary for complete psychological health (Bryant and Veroff 2007). In fact, the experience of spirituality may be an emotional one, inseparable from 'generalised good feelings'. Hence, positive emotions and a positive outlook as indices of mental health, and the experience of spiritual contact — of having glimpses of the divine — seem to be intimately related (Fredrickson 1998). When people feel the spiritual emotions that connect them to others, to society, to nature, and to the universe and beyond, they are likely to behave in a more balanced way, perhaps because they become better assessors of their typical existence in the world and the world around them. Mental health cannot slip into the mire of illness there.

From a humanistic and phenomenological perspective, Elkins et al. stated that 'spirituality', which comes from the Latin 'spiritus' meaning 'breath of life', is a 'way of being and experiencing that comes about through awareness of a transcendent dimension and that is characterized by certain identifiable values in regard to self, others, nature, life and whatever one considers to be the Ultimate' (1988: 10). At a behavioural level, the term spirituality is used to denote certain 'positive inward qualities and perceptions', while avoiding the implications of 'narrow dogmatic belief and obligatory religious observances' (Wulff 1996: 47). Spirituality, according to Emmons, 'encompasses a search for meaning, for unity, for connectedness, for transcendence, and for the highest of human potential' (1999: 92). According to Elkins et al. the major components of spirituality are:

1. A belief in the 'transcendental dimension' of experience as a 'greater self'.
2. Meaning and purpose in life.
3. A mission in life.
4. The sacredness of life.
5. Challenging material values.
6. Altruism or being affected by others' sufferings.
7. Idealism; having a vision of a better world.
8. Awareness of the tragic, i.e., that pain, sufferings and death are inevitable.
9. Fruits of spirituality; an improved relationship with oneself, nature and other human beings (1988: 33–35).

J. Swinton defined spirituality as

> an intra, inter and transpersonal experience that is shaped and directed by the experience of individuals and of the communities within which they live out their lives. It is 'intrapersonal' in having its quest for inner connectivity, 'interpersonal' in having relationships between people and within communities, and 'transpersonal' in so far as it reaches beyond self and others in the transcendent realms of experience (2001: 20).

Hence, the spiritual journey may be conceived as one of continuous learning, of purification, and of practically operationalising the implications of the same in mundane life.

The leaning towards spirituality is obvious today. The overarching human motivations are two-pronged: (*a*) to survive, and (*b*) to discover the meaning and purpose of survival. Individuals cannot long endure adversities and sufferings without a reason for living. Self-transcendence is essential to mental health and personal development, and spiritual coping seems to be an important aspect of adaptation. According to P. Dalby, some common spiritual themes in the advanced years of life are: 'integrity, humanistic concern, changing relationships with others, concern for younger generations, relationship with a transcendent being or power, self-transcendence and coming to terms with death' (2006: 4). Hence, spirituality 'speak[s] of inner empowerment, cultivating self-esteem, harvesting memories, transformative turning points, lifelong learning, themes of humour and gratitude and encountering morality' (Bianchi 2005).

In brief, spirituality is an exploration of the process of being involved in 'becoming fully human'. Personality orientations seem the most important factor in facilitating or hindering this process (West 2004). Of several factors having either a facilitative or inhibitory effect on spiritual inclination, and hence impacting mental health, 'perfectionism' has been found to have a double-edged influence. Therefore, the next sections attempt a further consideration of this specific trait in the context of mental health and spiritualism.

Perfectionism: The Interlink of Health and Ill-health in the Spiritualistic Pursuits of Life

The modern era is materialistic in its outlook. As discussed earlier, in the developmental stages of life, the parent–child relationship requires an adherence to rules and regulations. Given the contemporary demand for being successful in life and earning a distinctive 'identity' of their own, children are being pushed into the rat race of unhealthy competitiveness. To be competent and successful, one is expected to be 'perfect'. If the proper resources to mental health are available, some people may develop the right kind of adaptiveness for the perfectionism they seek. They may become organised and self-regulated in life. In other cases, much of such parental aspirational pressures result in high rates of guilt, a sense of failure, a sense of personal inadequacy, and an inability to achieve positive self-regard. They produce the maladaptive version of the perfectionist orientation, ultimately resulting in obsessive-compulsive traits in the personality along with morbid features of anxiety and depression. Since clinical evidence shows that the rate of obsession-compulsion in children is on the rise, research and theory on perfectionism has increased exponentially. According to G. L. Flett and P. L. Hewitt (2002), 336 publications with the term were published in the 1990s, as compared with 102 publications in the 1980s. Since this chapter attempts to point the way to psychological health through the elucidation of mental health in the wider context of spirituality, it is necessary to verify the role of 'perfectionism' as a personality correlate.

In a culture saturated with the emergence of self-help strategies, mostly for achieving success in terms of materialistic gains, perfectionist striving is bound to be obvious, because this variable serves as an important 'gearing force' in mobilising people's goal-oriented actions (Blatt 1995; Hollender 1978; Pacht 1984). The message is: No mistake is granted. Dimensionally, perfectionism has a 'normal' and a 'neurotic' bent. Normal perfectionism is defined as a striving for reasonable and realistic standards that lead to a sense of self-satisfaction and enhanced self-esteem; neurotic perfectionism is setting excessively high standards to be achieved, and is dogged by fears of failure and disappointment to others (Hamachek 1978). Using a different coinage, Terry-Short et al. describe 'positive perfectionism' as a reinforcer of positive behaviour, and 'negative perfectionism' as aversive responses to the challenges in life (1995: 663–68). Hence, perfectionism seems to have both 'adaptive' and 'maladaptive' versions. These 'two faces' of perfectionism serve as the 'interlink' between healthy lifestyles and realisation of transcendence on the one hand, and on the other, an excessive fear of God, anticipation of punishment and a bad name, losing one's identity altogether, and being immersed in dark patches of mental disorder, very far away from any kind of transcendental realisation and calmness of the self. Table 6.1 shows the mosaic patterns of these two dimensions of perfectionism in the mental health context.

Perfectionism: Its Interpersonal Aspects in Relation to Mental Health

The wealth of literature available to date demonstrates how perfectionism plays a key role in the experience of intrapersonal states such as depression, anxiety, and hopelessness. D. D. Burns and A. T. Beck (1978) discussed perfectionists' anticipated rejection and hypersensitivity to criticism as factors contributing to disturbed interpersonal relationships; this characteristic has been hypothesised to be related to a 'disclosure phobia' that promotes social withdrawal (Frost et al. 1995).

Interpersonal distress may be related to perfectionism in two ways. Perfectionism, whether self-directed or interpersonal, may affect relationships by working indirectly through promotion of intrapersonal pathology (Hewitt and Flett 1991; Ruscher and Gotlib 1988; Schmaling and Jacobson 1990). Or it may have direct effects on interpersonal relationships by limiting or impairing one's ability to interact in social

Table 6.1 Patterns of the Two Dimensions of Perfectionism

Maladaptive Perfectionism	*Adaptive Perfectionism*
• Unable to experience pleasure from labours	• Able to experience satisfaction or pleasure
• Inflexibly high standards	• Standards modified in accordance with the situation
• Unrealistically or unreasonably high standards	• Achievable standards
• Overly generalised high standards	• High standards are matched to the person's limitations and strengths
• Fear of failure	• Striving for success
• Focus on avoiding error	• Focus on doing things right
• Tense/anxious attitude towards tasks	• Relaxed but careful attitude
• Large gap between performance and standards	• Reasonable match between attainable performance and standards
• Sense of self-worth dependent on performance	• Sense of self-independence in performance
• Associated with procrastination	• Timely completion of tasks
• Motivation to avoid negative consequences	• Motivation to achieve positive feedback/rewards
• Goals attained for self-enhancement	• Goals attained for the enhancement of society
• Failure associated with harsh self-criticism	• Failure associated with disappointment and renewed efforts
• Black-and-white thinking: Perfection vs failure	• Balanced thinking
• Belief that one should excel	• Desire to excel
• 'Compulsive' tendencies and doubting	• Reasonable certainty about actions

contexts. For instance, perfectionists are likely to avoid relationships because of expectations of being hurt for failing to be perfect (Blatt 1995). Similarly, perfectionism may affect the quality of the relationships that are maintained, perhaps by stimulating aversive behaviours from others (Flett et al. 1997). Inquiry into the dynamics of maladaptive perfectionism also highlights the major role of self-conscious emotions — shame, guilt, embarrassment, and pride — which are fundamental emotions of evaluation, specifically with respect to the self. The perils of perfectionism are manifold. These, according to Mike Bellah (2011), are some of the important ones:

- Pride: Perfectionists come to believe that they are beyond failure. It keeps individuals from seeing the truth — that they do need forgiveness and they do need others.
- Phoniness: Perfectionists can never drop their guard, never relax, never just be themselves. It is a practice that, over time, causes identity problems.
- Pharisaism: Focusing on the shortcomings of others helps them feel good about themselves.
- Pettiness: Perfectionists forever strain out trivial things in life.
- Paranoia: Perfectionists have a hard time accepting friendship and love from others, for they tend to think that people are just waiting to catch them out in their imperfections.
- Paralysis: Perfectionism ultimately paralyses the perfectionist. They fail to achieve their personal best.

In its positive mode, perfectionism can be conducive to creating greater adaptive capacities and helping in achieving self-realisation. It is found to include:

- A relatedness (anaclitic)[1] developmental line, which leads to increasingly mature, mutually satisfying, reciprocal, interpersonal relationships.
- A self-definitional (introjective) developmental line, which leads to a consolidated, realistic, essentially positive, differentiated, and integrated identity.

The two developmental processes of relatedness and self-definition evolve throughout life in a reciprocal, mutually facilitating, dialectic transaction. An increasingly differentiated, integrated and mature sense of self emerges out of satisfying interpersonal relationships, resulting in the blossoming of the 'spiritual self' (Blatt 1990, 1995; Blatt and Blass 1990, 1996; Blatt and Shichman 1983). The self now acquires self-awareness and self-knowledge, and experiences an integrated meaning in life. It possesses certain 'positive inward qualities and perceptions' and encompasses a search for meaning, 'for unity', 'for connectedness', 'for transcendence', and 'for the highest of human potentials' (Pargament 1997). Self-transcendence, as mentioned, is essential to mental health and personal development, with spiritual coping appearing to be an important aspect of adaptation (Mc Nicol 1996; Pargament 1997). It can only be attained by the route of self-actualisation, which is propelled by the positive dimension of perfectionism. Hence, it is this dimension of perfectionism that enables an individual to embrace life through spiritual awareness, and helps foster mental health.

Conclusion

The objective world seems materialistic in its outer manifestations. To a growing child, concrete experiences are the root and route of learning in life. Yet, to make this world a beautiful and worthy place to live in, positive feelings and emotions need to be evoked by adults in the fresh and tender minds of children. Initially, a child needs role models to follow, to develop a self-regulated lifestyle, and to be able to inspire work-motivation and relationship development as life's key tasks for a healthy mental life. Gradually, by adopting an adaptive, positivistic, perfectionist approach to life, one attains self-realisation of a near, vision-focused reality, and after that into an inner reality of understanding things beyond concrete conception. This is the domain of spirituality, entry into which is essential for any true fulfilment of human life. Indeed, the seed of the true meaning of life is embedded there, with the assurance of 'no fear' and 'no anxiety' for those able to access it.

Note

1. According to Blatt et al. (2001), 'Anaclictic' patients are those who are excessively focused on relationship issues — including trust, intimacy and sexuality — whereas 'Introjective' patients are those focused on issues to do with the self, autonomy, self-worth and control.

References

Bellah, M. 2011. 'The Perils of Perfectionism', *Our Best Years: Home Page for 'Midlife Moments'*. Available at http://www.bestyears.com/perfectionism.html (accessed 30 September 2011).

Bianchi, E. 2005. Abstract of 'Living with Elder Wisdom', *Journal of Gerontological Social Work*, 45 (3): 319–29.

Blatt, S. J. 1990. 'Interpersonal Relatedness and Self-definition: Two Personality Configurations and Their Implications for Psychopathology and Psychotherapy', in J. L. Singer (ed.), *Repression and Dissociation: Implications for Personality Theory, Psychopathology and Health*, pp. 299–335. Chicago: University of Chicago Press.

———. 1995. 'Representational Structures in Psychopathology', in D. Ciccheti and S. Toth. Rochester (eds), *Rochester Symposium on Developmental Psychopathology: Vol 6. Emotion, Cognition, and Representation*, pp. 1–33. NY: University of Rochester Press.

Blatt, S. J. and R. B. Blass. 1990. 'Attachment and Separateness: A Dialectic Model of the Products and Processes of Psychological Development', *Psychoanalytic Study of the Child*, 45: 107–27.

———. 1996. 'Relatedness and Self-definition: A Dialectic Model of Personality Development', in G. C. Noam and K. W. Fisher (eds), *Development and Vulnerability in Close Relationships*, pp. 309–38. Hillsdale, NJ: Erlbaum.

Blatt, S. J., G. Shahar and D. C. Zuroff. 2001. 'Anaclitic (Sociotropic) and Introjective (Autonomous) Dimensions', *Psychotherapy*, 30 (4): 449–54.

Blatt, S. J. and S. Shichman. 1983. 'Two Primary Configurations of Psychopathology', *Psychoanalysis and Contemporary Thought*, 6: 167–254.

Bryant, F. B. and J. Veroff. 2007. *Savoring: A New Model of Positive Experience*. Mahwah, NJ: Lawrence Erlbaum.

Burns, D. D. and A. T. Beck. 1978. 'Cognitive Behaviour Modification of Mood Disorders', in J. P. Foreyt and D. P. Rathjen (eds), *Cognitive Behaviour Therapy*, pp. 109–34. New York: Plenum.

Dalby, P. 2006. 'Is There a Process of Spiritual Change or Development Associated with Ageing? A Critical Review of Research', *Ageing Mental Health*, 10 (1): 4–12.

Diener, E. and R. Biswas-Diener. 2008. *Happiness: Unlocking the Mysteries of Psychological Wealth*. Oxford: Blackwell Publishing.

Elkins, D. N., L. J. Hedstrom, L. L. Hughes, J. A. Leaf, and C. Saunders. 1988. 'Towards a Humanistic Phenomenological Spirituality: Definition, Description and Measurement', *Journal of Humanistic Psychology*, 28 (4): 5–18.

Emmons, Robert A. 1999. *Psychology of Ultimate Concerns*. New York: Guilford Press.

Flett, G. L. and P. L. Hewitt. 2002. 'Perfectionism and Maladjustment: An Overview of Theoretical, Definitional and Treatment Issues', in G. C. Flett and P. C. Hewitt (eds), *Perfectionism: Theory, Research and Treatment*, pp. 5–32. Washington: American Psychological Association.

Flett, G. L., P. L. Hewitt, M. Garshowitz, and T. R. Martin. 1997. 'Personality, Negative Social Interactions, and Depressive Symptoms', *Canadian Journal of Behavioural Science*, 29: 28–37.

Fredrickson, B. L. 1998. 'What Good Are Positive Emotions?', *Review of General Psychology*, 2: 300–19.

Frost, R. O., T. A. Turcotte, R. G. Heimberg, J. I. Mattia, C. S. Holt, and D. A. Hope. 1995. 'Reactions to Mistakes among Subjects High and Low in Perfectionistic Concern over Mistakes', *Cognitive Therapy and Research*, 19: 195–205.

Hamachek, D. E. 1978. 'Psychodynamics of Normal and Neurotic Perfectionism', *Psychology: A Journal of Human Behaviour*, 15: 27–33.

Hewitt, P. L. and G. L. Flett. 1991. 'Dimensions of Perfectionism in Unipolar Depression', *Journal of Abnormal Psychology*, 100: 98–101.

Hollender, M. H. 1978. 'Perfectionism: A Neglected Personality Trait', *Journal of Clinical Psychiatry*, 39: 384.

Keyes, C. 2002. 'The Mental Health Continuum: From Languishing to Flourishing in Life', *Journal of Health and Social Behaviour*, 43: 207–22.

Mc Nicol, T. 1996. 'The New Faith in Medicine', *USA Today*, 7 April, p. 4.

Pacht, A. R. 1984. 'Reflections on Perfection', *American Psychologist*, 39: 386–90.

Pargament, K. I. 1997. *The Psychology of Religion and Coping*. New York: Guilford Press.

Prince, M., V. Patel, S. Saxena, M. Maj, J. Maselko, M. R. Phillips, and A. Rahman. 2007. 'No Health without Mental Health', *Lancet*, 370 (9590): 859–77.

Rinpoche, S. 2008. *The Tibetan Book of Living and Dying: A Spiritual Classic From One of the Foremost Interpreters of Tibetan Buddhism to the West*. London: Rider.

Ruscher, S. M. and I. H. Gotlib. 1988. 'Marital Interaction Patterns of Couples With and Without a Depressed Partner', *Behaviour Therapy*, 19: 455–70.

Schmaling, K. B. and N. S. Jacobson. 1990. 'Marital Interaction and Depression', *Journal of Abnormal Psychology*, 99: 229–36.

Swinton, J. 2001. *Spirituality and Mental Health Care, Rediscovering a 'Forgotten' Dimension*. London, Philadelphia: Jessica Kingsley Publishers.

Terry-Short, L. A., R. G. Owens, P. D. Slade, and M. E. Dewey. 1995. 'Positive and Negative Perfectionism', *Personality and Individual Differences*, 18: 663–68.

Weare, K. 2000. *Promoting Mental, Emotional and Social Health: A Whole School Approach*. London: Routledge Falmer.

West, W. 2004. *Spiritual Issues in Therapy: Relating Experience to Practice*. New York: Palgrave Macmillan.

Witmer, J. M. and T. J. Sweeny. 1992. 'A Holistic Model for Wellness and Prevention over the Lifespan', *Journal of Counseling and Development*, 71: 140–48.

Wong, P. T. P. 2000. 'Meaning-centered Counselling Workshop', Paper presented at the International Conference on Searching for Meaning in the New Millennium, 13 July, Richmond, B. C.

World Health Organization. 2010. 'WHO | Mental Health: Strengthening our Response', *World Health Organization*, http://www.who.int/mediacentre/factsheets/fs220/en/ (accessed 30 September 2011).

Wulff, D. M. 1996. 'The Psychology of Religion: An Overview', in E. P. Shapraspse (ed.), *Religion and the Clinical Practice of Psychology*. Washington DC: American Psychological Association.

Seven

The Doctrine of the Three Humours in Traditional Indian Medicine

Hartmut Scharfe[1]

Siddha and Āyurveda

This study really began in 1968 at the Second World Tamil Conference in Madras, where the organisers had arranged for an exhibit of traditional Tamil medicine, with a large number of Siddha[2] practitioners present. Theirs was obviously an ancient art, and attempts have been made in recent decades to give it wider currency.[3] Just how old is Siddha medicine and how does it relate to the better known Ayurveda, since one can immediately see that they have much in common and are practiced side by side in south India? My interest was aroused, as one who had strayed from the family profession of medicine, and I felt an urge to bring light to this mystery of medical history.

Almost from the beginning I was confronted with conflicting claims put forth in the strongest terms. Tamil practitioners tend to insist on the highest antiquity for their tradition, whereas V. Raghavan, the noted Sanskrit scholar, once told me years ago that Siddha medicine is nothing but a derivative of Āyurveda. If one views these claims against the background of tension persisting between the propagandists of Tamil culture, on the one hand, and brahmins (even Tamil brahmins), on the other, which has marked much of this century, one might be tempted to reject both claims as biased. But the claim of Āyurveda is backed by one obvious trump card: the terminology of Siddha medicine is overwhelmingly based on Sanskrit. Siddha texts speak of the three *tātu* or *tōcam*, i.e., *vāta*, *pittam*, and *cilēṭṭumam*, undeniably Tamil reflections of Sanskrit *dhātu*, *doṣa*, *vāta*, *pitta*, and *śleṣman*, as the basic constituents of the body; the same is true for much of the anatomical vocabulary: *kāyam* 'body', nāḍī 'nerve, artery', *nayana* 'eye' are found even in the titles of various Siddha texts, such as *Kāya-kaṟpa*, *Nāḍī-nūl*, *Nayana-viti*.

One Siddha practitioner countered (in conversation) with the argument that it was fashionable for many centuries to replace old Tamil names and terms with more 'prestigious' Sanskrit expressions, just as we see a replacement of the old place names Ciṟṟampalam (frequently in the 7th-century *Tēvāram*; e.g., at 1.1) or Tillai (*Tiruvācakam* 8.5) with today's Citamparam (Chidambaram);[4] older Kuṭantai and Kūṭa-mūkku 'Pot-nose' by Kumpakōṇam (i.e., Kumbha-ghoṇa).[5] Still, it would be difficult to accept such a massive change of terminology in a medicine that — at least in minds and statements of contemporary practitioners[6] — prides itself in being distinctively Tamil.

Several authors have attempted to demonstrate the high antiquity of Siddha medicine by alleged references to Siddha practices in the old Sangam literature.[7] We can see that these references to human anatomy and certain treatments indicate that two thousand years ago the Tamils had knowledge of and names for certain parts of the human body (who would have doubted that?) and that they knew of some practices of treatment and healing. The word *maruntu* 'medicine, medication' is common in the Sangam poems, and there are references to medical men *maruttuvaṉ* (pl. *maruttuvar*); two poets have the word attached to their names: Maruttuvaṉ Tāmōtaraṉār (i.e., Dāmodara)[8] and Maruttuvaṉ Nallaccutaṉār.[9] Some form of medical practice can probably be found in any society, but there is nothing that points specifically to the practice of Siddha or of Āyurveda medicine in the time of the Sangam poetry.

The first reference to Āyurveda is found in *Cilappatikāram* V.44, where *āyuḷvētar* 'experts in Āyurveda' are said to live in the centre of town next to priests and astrologers.[10] The *Cilappatikāram* is one of the later Sangam texts and is now tentatively dated by K. Zvelebil to about A.D. 450.[11] Still later, probably, is the *Tirukkuṟaḷ*,[12] which states in stanza 941: 'The three, having wind (*vaḷi*) as first, as they (i.e., these three)[13] increase or diminish, will cause disease (*noy*)'.This is an obvious reference to the wind, bile, and phlegm that play a crucial role in the pathology of both Siddha medicine and Āyurveda. But the poet used no comprehensive term for this triad — neither the word *doṣa* nor any of its Tamil equivalents that we find in typical Siddha texts.

The oldest existing Siddha text is the *Tirumantiram*,[14] whose date scholars have tried to establish through elaborate investigations of who quotes or refers to whom. Does a reference in *Tirumantiram* 1646 (1619) to the five *maṇḍala*s of the Tamil country point to an early date?[15] Does Sundaramūrti (9th century) in his *Tiruttoṇḍa-ttokai* (5.5) refer to the author of the *Tirumantiram* when he mentions a certain Tirumūlar? Based on how a scholar evaluates these references, the estimated date varies from the 5th century A.D.[16] to the 11th century. A reference to the nine Nāthasiddhas in *Tirumantiram* 3067[17] and the description of the concepts of the Buddhist Kālacakra school in section III, chapter 14[18] are taken by R. Venkatraman[19] as an indication that this text belongs to the 10th or 11th century and that its author, Tirumūlar, must be distinguished from the Tirumūlar mentioned by Sundaramūrti.[20] We must also consider the possibility that our text of the *Tirumantiram* contains later additions.[21] The earliest clear reference to the *Tirumantiram* is found in a 12th-century work, Sēkkiḻār's *Tiruttoṇḍar Purāṇam*.[22] A commentary (11th or 12th century?) on the *Yāpparutkalam* quotes *Tirumantiram* 204 (247), with slight variations.[23]

The exact dating of the *Tirumantiram* is of minor importance in the present context, because the text contains no specific references to Siddha medical doctrines.[24] There is no mention of diagnostics by feeling the pulse,[25] the pharmacological use of heavy metals,[26] or even the theory of the three *tōca*, though wind, bile, and phlegm as the cause of trouble are known (see later in chapter).

The bulk of the texts associated with the thought and medicine of the Siddhas appears to be much later. Two Siddha scholars[27] readily admitted to me that the language of these rather voluminous texts is late, probably nŏt older than the 16th century A.D., and R. Venkatraman's investigations of these works and the legends connected with the names of their presumed authors confirm this — but could these works be the written reflections of an oral tradition that goes back to a hoary past? Or, to put it in another way, between the two competing medical systems — Siddha and Āyurveda — which way did the borrowing go?

The key to the solution of this problem is, I think, the presumed role of the three faults or humours in man's physical well-being common to contemporary Siddha and Āyurveda medicines. In modern times we read and hear of *tiridoṣam* or *tiritōcam*, simple adaptations of a Sanskrit *tri-doṣam* to Tamil phonology. *Muttōcam* replaces Sanskrit *tri* 'three' with the Tamil equivalent *mū* (with shortening of the/ū/in composition). Older — and more problematic — is *mu-kkuṟṟam* 'the three evils' of the soul in Nālaḍiyār 190 (7th century?), i.e., *kāmam* 'desire', *vekuḷi* 'anger', and *mayakkam* 'confusion'[28] which apparently have no medical connotations. The three blemishes (*mūṉ ṟruḷa kuṟ ṟam*) in *Tirumantiram* 2435f. (2396f.) are lust, anger, and ignorance — also ethical, not medical problems. *Mu-kuṟṟam* would thus be similar to *mu-mmalam* 'three impurities' in *Tirumantiram* 343 (329), i.e., 'egoity, karma, maya' in the words of B. Natarajan. Notice in contrast the different terminology, when in *Tirumantiram* 727 (707) yoga practiced at dusk is said to remove phlegm (*ai*);[29] at noon, the treacherous wind (*vāta*); at dawn, bile (*pitta*) — allowing the yogin to escape old age. Here phlegm, wind, and bile are all seen as evils to be gotten rid of, as in some medical texts; and yet no general term, such as 'three evils', is used for phlegm, wind, and bile. *Tirumantiram* 458 (442)[30] refers to a balance of qualities that is beneficial for an infant, but I very much doubt that this is a reference to the 'balance of the *doṣas*'. Only in more recent Siddha texts, it seems[31] — and in contemporary writings[32] — we are told that health is based on a balance of the three 'faults' or 'evils', i.e., wind, bile, and phlegm. In contemporary usage, these three, called *tiri-tōṣam* or *mu-ttōṣam* 'three faults' or *mu-ppiṇi* 'three maladies'[33] are supposed to be balanced for good health. These three are often referred to in English writings (on both schools of traditional Indian medicine) as the three 'humo(u)rs', as if this term[34] made their role in maintaining good health more acceptable. The introduction of the term is caused by an insidious side-glance at Greek medicine, where the four humours (the word used is χυμοί 'juices')[35] — blood, phlegm, yellow bile, and black bile[36] — play a central role in the texts of the hippocratic corpus (perhaps rather in the younger texts of this corpus). There is yet another reason why the term is ill-suited to Indian medicine as a common term for wind, bile, and phlegm: wind is obviously not a fluid or 'humor' in the ordinary sense of the word. Use of the term in any discussion of Indian medicine creates the doubtful presumption of a similarity to or even a dependence on the Greek medical tradition, which could at best, perhaps, be established as a result of a thorough investigation.

It seems strange that positive well-being should be based on a balance of evils; one would at least like to see an explanation for this peculiar way of looking at things. A survey of the Tamil tradition fails to turn up convincing evidence of how the view evolved, but the late attestation of the *tri-doṣa* theory in Tamil medicine may offer a clue. The seemingly odd expression could have been borrowed from a tradition where its evolution was more meaningful. In the following pages I shall try to show that this was, in fact, the case. The theory of the three 'faults'as fundamental to health and illness evolves, as it were, under the influence of philosophical ideas that were current at the time the classical medical texts were composed or redacted. We shall now turn our attention to the north Indian tradition.

The Evidence of the Buddhist Canon

There are several references in the Buddhist canon to wind, bile, and phlegm as causes of illness; the term *doṣa* is also found in the canonical texts, but wind, bile, and phlegm are, as such, never so identified, either individually or jointly, and no reference to a *tri-doṣa* theory occurs. Since the illnesses and their cures described in the canon have been discussed in detail by Kenneth G. Zysk in a recent book,[37] I shall limit myself here to a short presentation of the relevant passages. At the risk of appearing repetitive, I will have to review some of Zysk's key evidence to show the use of important terms and to justify my critique of his translation of the term *doṣa* in the Pali texts.

Aṅguttara-nikāya IV.320:

> *so mama assa antarāyo. upakkhalitvā vd papateyyaṃ, bhattaṃ vā me bhuttaṃ byāpajjeyya, pittaṃ vā me kuppeyya, semhaṃ vā me kuppeyya, satthakā vā me vātā kuppeyyuṃ, manussā vā maṃ upakkameyyu, amanussā vā maṃ upakkameyyuṃ; tena me assa kālaṅkiriyā.*
>
> This may be my death: I may stumble and fall, the food I have eaten may kill me, my bile may get angry, my phlegm may get angry, my cutting winds may get angry, men may attack me, demons may attack me; in this way my end may come.

Aṅguttara-nikāya V.218 (cf., also V.219):

> *tikicchakā, bhikkhave, virecanaṃ denti pitta-samutthā nānaṃ pi ābādhānaṃ paṭighātāya, semha-samutthānānaṃ pi abddhdnaṃ patighātāya, vāta-samutthānānaṃ pi ābādhānaṃ paṭighātāya.*

O monks, physicians give a purgative as a cure for diseases that arise from bile, as a cure for diseases that arise from phlegm, as a cure for diseases that arise from wind.

Mahāvagga VI.14.1 + 3f. (Vinaya 1.205)

tena kho pana samayena āyasmato Pilindavacchassa vātābādho hoti . . .

Again, at that time the venerable Pilindavaccha had affliction of wind . . .

tena kho pana samayena āyasmato Pilindavacchassa anga-vāto hoti . . .

Again, at that time the venerable Pilindavaccha had wind in the limbs . . . [rheumatism?]

tena kho pana samayena āyasmato Pilindavacchassa pabba-vāto hoti . . .

Again, at that time the venerable Pilindavaccha had wind in the joints . . . [intermittent ague?]

Mahāvagga VI.16.3 (Vinaya 1.210; cf., also VI.17.1)

tena kho pana samayena aññatarassa bikkhuno udaravātâbādho hoti.

Again, at that time a certain monk had affliction of wind in the abdomen.

Saṃyutta-nikāya IV.230f., lists the eight determining causes, beginning with phlegm, bile, wind, and their combination:

pitta-samutthānāni pi kho, Sīvaka, idhekaccāni vedayitāni uppajjanti. sāmaṃ pi kho etaṃ, Sīvaka, veditabbam
yathā pitta-samutthānāni pi idhekaccāni vedayitāni uppajjanti;
lokassa pi kho etaṃ, Sīvaka, sacca-sammataṃ
yathā pitta-samutthānāni pi idhekaccāni vedayitāni uppajjanti. . .
semha-samutthānāni pi kho. . .
vāta-samutthānāni pi kho . . .

sannipātikāni pi kho . . .
utu-pariṇāma-jāni pi kho . . .
pittaṃ semhaṃ ca vāto ca, sannipātā utūni ca /
visamam opakkamikaṃ ca, kamma-vipākena ammhamī ti / /

Now, Sīvaka, in this connection, there are some sufferings originating from bile. You ought to know by experience, Sīvaka, that this is so. And this fact, that sufferings originate from bile, is generally acknowledged by the world as true . . .
Also originating from phlegm . . .
Also originating from wind . . .
Also originating from their combination . . .
Also originating from changes of the season . . .
Bile, phlegm, and wind, their combination and the seasons, mishaps and foreign impact, together with the ripening of one's karma: that is eight.[38]

The same list of eight causes is found also in *Aṅguttaranikāya* II.87 and III.131. Note that *sannipāta* 'combination' implies a close connection of the preceding three items: bile, phlegm, and wind. As these three are not identified in canonical texts as the three *doṣa*s, there is no justification for Demiéville to speak of a 'theory of four humors — wind, phlegm, bile and the combination of the three'.[39]

In *Mahāvagga* VIII.1.30–33 (*Vinaya* I.278f.) Buddha's body is said to be flooded with *doṣa*s:

atha kho Bhagavato kāyo dosābhisanno hoti . . .

At that time the body of the Blessed one was flooded with faults . . .

The famous physician Jīvaka Komārabhacca gave him a mild purgative. The same affliction is apparently meant in *Mahāvagga* VI.14.7 (*Vinaya* I.206):[40]

tena kho pana samayena aññataro bhikkhu abhisannakāyo hoti.

Again, at that time a certain monk had a flooded body.

He, too, is given a purgative. His body was flooded, we may assume, with faults — as in the previous quotation. The phrase has a parallel in *Caraka-saṃhitā*, Kalpasthāna, 12:8:

pibet gulmôdarī doṣair abhikhinnaś ca yo naraḥ
go-mṛgâja-rasaiḥ pāṇḍuḥ kṛmi-koṣṭhī bhagandarī

A man with an abdominal tumor and one attacked by the faults, one who is pale, who has a belly of worms, one who has a fistula-in-ano should drink [. . .] with juice of cow's, deer's or goat's [meat]

with a variant reading *abhiṣyaṇṇaś ca yo naraḥ*, which would correspond well with Pali *abhisanna*. Forms of the root *syand* with the prefix *abhi* are well attested, whereas there is no trace of any other form of the root *khid* with *abhi*.

The faults or corruptions (Pali *dosa*, Sanskrit *doṣa*) refer, in the classical medical texts, usually to wind, bile, and phlegm as the cause of illnesses. The same might be presumed to be the case here, too; but there is no clear instance of such usage in the Pali texts.[41] It is also not known whether *abhisanna-kāyo* is an abbreviated version of *dosâbhisannna-kāyo* or the latter an elaboration based on later ideas. The relative chronology of the Pali passages quoted cannot at present be ascertained, and the whole Kalpasthāna of the *Carakasaṃhitā* is the work of the redactor Dṛḍhabala (8th century?).

I have to take issue here with Zysk's translation of *doṣa* from the canonical passages (and from *Caraka*) as '"peccant" humors'.[42] Not only is the expression 'humor' misleading, as I pointed out earlier, but the qualification 'peccant' surreptitiously affirms the negative aspect required by the context. If the word *doṣa* 'humor' is value-neutral, why do we not see any 'good' *doṣas* in the Pali canon (or in *Caraka*, for that matter)? Zysk rightly stresses the continuity between early Buddhist and early Āyurvedic medicine, in that wind, bile, and phlegm — or a combination of these — are causes of many ailments, though in several instances ailments are not traced to any of these three.[43] But he treads on thin ice when he concludes that the textual evidence 'does not imply the absence of humoral etiology at this time'.[44] In fact, it doesn't imply its presence either, as R. Müller pointed out many years ago.[45] *Doṣa* in these cases rather seems to denote something that should not normally be there in the body, a 'fault', possibly referring to abnormal conditions of wind, bile, and phlegm. Still, this would be far from what is usually understood by a 'humoral etiology'.

In a few other occurrences of the word, *doṣa* is used in a more general sense.[46] In *Mahāvagga* VI. 14.7 (*Vinaya* 1.206):

tena kho pana samayena aññatarassa bhikkhuno chavidosâbādho hoti

Again, at that time a certain monk had an affliction of skin corruption

chavi-dosa corresponds to classical *tvag-doṣa* 'corruption of the skin, skin disease', found in *Caraka*, Sūtra-sthāna, 3.29; *Bhela*, Sūtra-sthāna, 6.17; and *Suśruta*, Sūtra-sthāna, 24.10 and Cikitsita-sthāna, 9.1f.

There are several lists of body parts in the Buddhist canon and in the preceding Vedic literature[47] that include, besides the more obvious bones and organs, bile and phlegm. The oldest detailed lists are probably those found in the brāhmaṇa sections of the saṃhitās of the Black Yajurveda: *Taittirīya-saṃhitā* V.7.11–23 (14 *prāṇa* 'breath'; 20 *dūṣīkā* 'rheum of the eyes'; 23 *pitta* 'bile'); cf.,*Maitrāyaṇi-saṃhitā* III.15.1ff. (2 *prāṇa*, 8 *dūṣīkā*, 9 *pitta*) and *Kāṭhaka-saṃhitā* 53 (10 *dūṣīkā*, 12 *pitta*). A similar list is found, in the White Yajurveda, in *Vājasaneyi-saṃhitā* XXV. 1–9 (2 *prāṇāḥ*, 7 *pitta*, 9 *dūṣīkā*).

In the Buddhist canon, *Dīgha-nikāya* II.293f. has the following list:[48]

puna ca paraṃ, bhikkhave, bhikkhu imam eva kāyaṃ,
uddhaṃ pādatalā adho kesa-matthakā, taca-pariyantaṃ
pūraṃ nānappakārassaa sucino paccavekkhati: atthi imasmiṃ
kāye kesā lomā nakhā dantā taco maṃsam nhāru aṭṭhi
aṭṭhimiñjaṃ vakkaṃ hadayaṃ yakanaṃ kilomakaṃ pihakam
papphāsaṃ antaṃ antaguṇaṃ udariyaṃ karīsaṃ
pittaṃ semhaṃ pubbo lohitaṃ sedo medo assu vasā kheḷo
siṅghanikā lasikā muttaṃ ti . . .
puna ca paraṃ, bhikkhave, bhikkhu imam eva kāyaṃ
yathāṭhitaṃ yathāpaṇihitaṃ dhātuso paccavekkhati: atthi
imasmiṃ kāye pathavī-dhātu, āpo-dhātu, tejo-dhātu,
vāyo-dhātū ti.

Furthermore, O monks, the monk views this body, from the feet upward and from the hair and the head downward, up to the skin filled with various impurities: In this body there are hair of the head, hair of the body, nails, teeth, skin, flesh, sinews, bones, bone marrow, kidneys, heart, liver, pleura, spleen, lungs, bowels, intestines, stomach, excrement, bile, phlegm, pus, blood, sweat, fat, tears, grease, saliva, mucus, serous fluid, and urine . . . Furthermore, O monks, the monk views this body as it stood, as it was put together from elements: There is in this body earth element, water element, fire element, and wind element.

To sum up: it is clear that bile and phlegm were considered in Buddhist doctrine as part of the human body even (unexpelled) faeces and urine. Breath, however is not included.[49] *Doṣas* cause illness, but nothing more is said about them.

The Evidence in the *Mahābhāṣya*[50]

Pāṇini V.1.38 [18 *ṬHaⁿ*]*tasya nimittaṃ saṃyogōtpātau* '[The suffix-ika is attached to denote that this is] its effective purpose, provided that a conjunction or an omen is meant'. [E.g., if one associates with a rich man in order to borrow a hundred rupees (*śata*), that man may be termed 'worth a hundred' (*śātika*).]

Kātyāyana wants to expand the rule:

> *tasya-nimitta-prakaraṇe vāta-pitta-śleṣmabhyaḥ*
> *śamana-kopanayor upasaṃkhyānam*
>
> Under the topic "its effective purpose", [the meanings] "calming"and "riling", must be additionally enumerated, [when the suffix] follows [the words] *vāta* 'wind', *pitta* 'bile', or *śleṣman* 'phlegm'.

Patañjali paraphrases the *vārttika* and exemplifies it:

> *vātasya sámanaṃ kopanaṃ vā vātikam; paittikam; ślaiṣmikam.*
>
> [A medicine or procedure] that serves to calm or rile wind (*vāta*) is termed a 'wind-calmant' or a 'wind-rilant' [procedure] (*vātika*); one that serves to calm or rile bile is termed a 'bile-calmant' or 'bile-rilant' [procedure]; one that serves to calm or rile phlegm is termed a 'phlegmcalmant' or 'phlegm-rilant' [procedure].

Kātyāyana further expands the rule:

> *saṃnipātāc ca*
>
> And [when the suffix] follows [the word] *saṃnipāta*.

Patañjali explains:

> *saṃnipātāc cêti vaktavyam: sāṃnipātikam*

> [A medicine or procedure] that serves to calm or rile a combination (*saṃnipāta*) of wind, bile, or phlegm] is termed a 'combinatory-calmant' or a 'combinatory-rilant' [procedure] (*sāṃnipātika*).

This passage of the *Mahābhāṣya* shows the same group of wind, bile, and phlegm plus their combination, called *saṃnipāta*, that we found in the Pali canon as causes of illness and, as in that canon, they are not linked to the term *doṣa*.[51] In the Pali text it is said that wind/bile/phlegm *kupyate* 'gets angry'; Katāyāna speaks of riling them (*kopana*). The adjectives *vātika*, *paittika*, and *ślaiṣmika* for illnesses caused by *vāta*, *pitta*, and *śleṣman* are common in medical texts; but there are no unambiguous instances where they mean 'riling *vāta*, *pitta*, or *śleṣman*', and only rarely do we find *vātika* 'removing/calming wind'.[52] Since Kātyāyana can be dated to around 250 B.C. and Patañjali to 150 or 120 B.C., they are roughly contemporary with the works of the Buddhist canon, and their expressions are compatible with those found in the canon. Though Kātyāyana and Patañjali share the expressions *vātika*, *paittika*, *ślaiṣmika*, and *sāṃnipātika* with the classical medical texts, the meanings of these terms do not match exactly with those found in the medical texts and may represent a different strain of tradition, showing perhaps a regional/dialectal difference.

To sum up: the evidence is similar to that of the Buddhist canon, but *doṣa* is not mentioned. The terms *vātika*, *paittika*, *ślaiṣmika*, and *sāṃnipātika* are similar if not identical in meaning with those in the classical medical texts.

The Bower Manuscript and Contemporary Buddhist Texts

The Bower manuscript,[53] found in eastern Turkestan, has been placed, for paleographical reasons, in the time between the 4th and 6th century A.D.; current research favours the period between the beginning and the middle of the 6th century.[54] The manuscript contains several Buddhist texts, three of them dealing with medicine, which may be considerably older than the surviving manuscript.

The first text deals with the medicinal use of garlic, which 'removes the strength of wind' (15 *pavana-balaharaḥ*), 'calms bile' (15 *pitta-praśamanaḥ*), and 'defeats the strength of phlegm' (15 *kapha-bala-vijayī*), i.e., 'it removes the triad of faults' (15 *doṣa-traya-haraḥ*).[55] Sometimes the expressions are stronger: garlic 'kills the wind' (16 *pavanaṃ vinihanti*), certain drinks 'remove bile and phlegm' (49 *pitta-kaphâpahāḥ*), a certain medicine 'removes bile, blood, and wind' (85 *pittâsravātâpaham*) or just bile and blood (80 *vāta-raktâpaham*), wind and phlegm (82 *vāta-kaphāpaham*) or the faults (92 *doṣāpahān*, 120 *doṣa-harāḥ*). These expressions might be explained as merely emphatic exaggerations, or by attraction in mixed formulations like this: garlic 'kills tumor (caused) by wind if joined with (other) wind-killers' (38 *hanyād yukto māruta-gulmaṃpavana-ghnaiḥ*). Killing a tumour is unobjectionable; killing one's wind, however, is questionable.

These actions against wind, bile, and phlegm are important because the three cause illness. We learn about 'eye disease caused by wind' (70 *vāta-kṛte' kṣi-roge*), 'eye diseased caused by bile or blood' (73 *paitte' kṣi-roge rudhirâtmake ca*), and 'eye disease caused by phlegm' (76 *śleṣma-kṛte' kṣi-roge*), and 'coughing caused by wind' (121 *māruta-kāsinam*, 124; *vāta-kāsa* 129–31) as well as 'coughing caused by bile' (132 *paittike* [*kāse*]).

The role of blood in this context is curious, as it seems to join wind, bile, and phlegm as a cause of illness that has to be removed.[56] While one might argue that phlegm and wind are undesirable intruders (phlegm was not listed as part of the body in the older Vedic ritual texts, though it was in the *Śatapatha-brāhmaṇa* and in Buddhist texts), this cannot be said about bile, which has always been considered part of a healthy body (only healthy animals[57] could be part of a Vedic sacrifice), and certainly not about blood. The ambiguous role of blood — often lining up with the *doṣa*s while frequently listed as one of the bodily elements (*dhātu*) — has been discussed by several later Āyurvedic authors.[58]

'Phlegm together with wind . . . goes into anger' (101 *śleṣmā sa-vāyuḥ . . . prakopaṃyāti*), and garlic 'calms phlegm that is not long established' (16 *kapham apy acirād uditaṃ śamayet*); there is a 'calming of the illnesses caused by phlegm, blood, bile, and wind' (108 *kaphâsra-pittânila-roga-śāntau*). The contrast of *prakopa* and *śamayet / śānti* reminds us of Kātyāyana's vārttika *kopana-śamanayoḥ*. The combination of two such causes is called *saṃsarga*; of all three (blood was probably not included), probably **sarva-samutthāna*; thus diseases caused by two are called *saṃ sarga-ja* and those caused by all *sarva-samutthita* (78).

The ideal state is 'the balance of the elements' (44 *dhātūnāṃ sāmyam*), for 'health derives from the balance of the elements' (45 *dhātu-sāmyād ārogyam*). What are these elements? One might think of the four elements earth, water, fire, and wind that we found in the list in the Buddhist canon. But it is more likely that the elements meant here are the seven elements listed in the classical medical texts (*Car* Śa 6.10; *Suś* Sū 14.10f.): chyle, blood, flesh, fat, bone, marrow, and semen. Or, they could be the three elements wind, bile, and phlegm.

The second text in the Bower manuscript is the *Nāvanītakam* 'Made from Butter', essentially an Āyurvedic formulary for the treatment of various illnesses. We read about 'tumor caused by wind' (79 *vāta-kṛtaṃ ca gulmam*), 'tumor (caused) by an excess of wind or phlegm' (32 *gulme vāta-kaphōlbaṇe*), 'tumor (caused) by bile' (154 *pitta-gulma-*), and so on. Diseases in general can be 'caused by any of these: wind, blood, bile, phlegm, and their combination' (308f. *vāta-jān rogān*, *rakta-jān*, *pitta-jān*, *śleṣmikān*, *saṃnipātôtthān*). Such 'diseases caused by a combination (of causes)' are called *rogā ye sāṃnipātikāḥ* (250), using a term already demanded by Kātyāyana and made explicit by Patañjali. Note that here *sāṃnipātika* seems to include diseases caused by blood as if it were a fourth fault or cause.

It is not clear what is meant by the expression 'when the elements are broken apart by wind' (358 *vāta-bhagnecu dhātuṣu*); the elements (*dhātu*) should again be the classical constituents of the body, which are disturbed in some way. The opposite process is obviously envisioned in the phrase 'when the fault is removed (and) the elements settled' (385 *hṛte doṣe viprasannecu dhātuṣu*). Here the 'fault' (*doṣa*) is clearly not among the 'elements' (*dhātu*).

As illness is caused by the three (or even four?) faults, the cure consists in combatting the faults and their effects. A certain medical powder 'pushes off the combination [of the faults]' (58 *saṃnipāta-nud*); another treatment 'pushes off phlegm and wind' (156 *kapha-vāta-nud*), another 'strikes down wind' (185 *vātaṃ nihanti*). The cure is often seen as the calming of the disease or the causal fault: 'calming of all diseases' (288 *sarva-vyādhipraśamanam*), 'calming of wind and blood' (*vāta-śoṇitapraśamanam*, the colophon after 405, refers back to *vatā-rakta-haram* 'removing wind and blood' in 405), 'calming of all fevers' (501 *sarva-jvarāṇāṃ śamanaḥ*). This text seems to use *śamana* and *praśamana* without distinction; the former matches Kātyāyana's usage, the latter the usage of the classical texts.

The third medical text of the Bower manuscript offers little for our study except some medical terms postulated by Kātyāyana and exemplified by Patañjali: 47 *vātikā vṛṣaṇā* (*ḥ*) ('testes with wind') and

50 *śleṣmikā rogāvātikāḥ paittikāś ca* ('illnesses caused by phlegm, wind, and bile'). But the adjectives *vātika*, etc., do not have quite the meaning envisioned by Kātyāyana, i.e., 'riling/calming wind, etc'.[59] There is also a slight deviation in the form *śleṣmika* found here and in the *Nāvanītaka*; the correct form should be *ślaiṣmika* with *vṛddhi* in the first syllable, as demanded in the *Mahābhāṣya*.

There is also a two-page fragment of a medical text from Turkestan, edited by H. Lüders[60] and dated around A.D. 200 on palaeographical grounds. It contains several references to wind, bile, and phlegm, and may perhaps represent a development of medicine similar to that found in the Bower manuscript.

In Aśvaghoṣa's *Buddhacarita* III.42f., the charioteer explains the shocking appearance of a sick man to the young prince Siddhārtha: 'Friend, a great misfortune called disease has grown, arisen from the anger of the constituents (*dhātu-prakopa-prabhavaḥ*), by which even this strong man is made helpless'.[61] The young Siddhārtha asks further: 'Has this fault (*doṣa*) come into being separately for him alone, (or) is there a general danger of disease for (all)men?' It looks as if *dhātu* here refers to wind, bile, and phlegm as constituents of the body, and *doṣa* probably refers to any one of these as it has been riled; it is not impossible, though, that *doṣa* could refer to the man's diseased state itself.

In *Buddhacarita* X.20, in a formal exchange of courtesies, the king inquires about (his guest's) 'evenness of constituents' (*dhātu-sāmyam*). The guest, in turn, asks with equal kindness about the king's 'mental well-being and his (physical) health' (*manaḥ-svāsthyam anāmayaṃ ca*). The same formalities are expressed thus in *Buddhacarita* XII.3:

> *tāv ubhau nyāyataḥ pṛṣṭvā dhātu-sāmyaṃ parasparam*
>
> After both had properly asked each other about their evenness of constituents [i.e., their health]

In *Suvarṇaprabhāsasūtra* 16.3f., Jalavāhana asks his father, the medical doctor Jaṭiṃdhara:

> How is medicine to be practiced in order to cure a disease
> when it has arisen due to wind, bile, phlegm, or a combination
> (of these)? At what time is wind disturbed, at
> what time is bile disturbed, at what time is phlegm disturbed,
> so that men are oppressed?

From his father's response, note stanza 9:

> Illnesses duc to excess of wind occur in the rainy season. Disturbance of the bile takes place in autumn. Likewise, (illness) due to a combination (arises) in winter-time. Illnesses due to excess of phlegm arise in the hot season.[62]

Although the term *doṣa* is not found in this chapter, phlegm, bile, and wind are referred to as the 'triad of elements' (*dhātu-tritaya*) in stanza 11, and their being angered (*dhātu-tritaya-prakopaḥ*) is a sequential affair: 'Excess of phlegm erupts as soon as one has eaten. Excess of bile erupts during digestion. Excess of wind erupts as soon as one has digested'.[63]

To sum up: we found in this group of texts a 'triad of faults' (*doṣa-traya*), a 'triad of elements' (*dhātu-tritaya*), and good health defined as the 'balance of the elements' (*dhātu-sāmya*). The elements (*dhātu-*) are settled or serene when the faults (*doṣa*) are removed; these faults appear to be various states of wind, bile, and phlegm.

The *Caraka-saṃhitā*

The *Caraka-saṃhitā* presents itself as Caraka's redaction[64] of Agniveśa's work, but the bulk of book VI (Cikitsā-sthānam) and the books VII (Kalpa-sthānam) and VIII (Siddhi-sthānam) were added much later by Dṛḍhabala (approximately 8th century A.D.) as a replacement for lost portions of the text.[65] It is probable that the whole text has been subjected to some amount of rewriting by Dṛḍhabala.[66] I shall first take up the material found in book one (Sūtra-sthānam).

The goal of medicine is defined thus in Sūtra-sthāna 1.53:

> *kāryaṃ dhātu-sāmyam ihôcyate*
> *dhātu-sāmya-kriyā côktā tantrasyâsya prayojanam*
>
> In the present context, the effect is the equilibrium of [body] constituents. The very object of this science is the maintenance of the equilibrium of [body] constituents.

A similar statement is offered in Sūtra-sthāna 16.34:

> *yābhiḥ kriyābhir jāyante śarīre dhātavaḥ samāḥ*
> *sā cikitsā vikārāṇāṃ karma tad bhicajāṃsmṛtam*

Such actions by which balanced constituents arise in the
Body — these constitute treatment of diseases; that is considered
the duty of physicians.

What are these constituents? They could be the seven *dhātu* mentioned in *Śārīra-sthāna* 6.10, but they could also be wind, bile, and phlegm, as the following stanzas suggest (Sūtra-sthāna 7.39–41):

sama-pittânila-kaphāḥ kecid garbhâdi mānavāḥ
dṛśyante vātalāḥ kecit pittalāḥ ślecmalās tathā
teṣām anāturāḥ pūrve, vātalâdyāḥ sadâturāḥ
doṣânuśayitā hy eṣāṃ deha-prakṛtir ucyate
viparīta-guṇas teṣāṃ svastha-vṛtter vidhir hitaḥ
sama-sarva-rasaṃ sâtmyaṃ sama-dhātoḥ praśasyate

Some persons have the equilibrium of bile, wind, and
phlegm from the very time of conception; some are dominated
by wind, some by bile, some by phlegm. Of these,
the first are healthy, those dominated by wind, etc., are
always bound to get sick; their body constitution is named
after the fault [that afflicts them]. A prescription [of diet
and regimen] for their healthy life is laid down that has
the opposite qualities [of the dominant constituent that
gives them trouble]. For persons having balanced constituents,
habitual intake of diets consisting of all tastes
in proportionate quantity is prescribed.

Here wind, bile, and phlegm are called *dhātu* 'constituent' in stanza 41; ideally they are in balance.[67] If one of them is found in excess, it is called a *doṣa*, and the person thus afflicted is called *vātala* 'dominated by wind', *pittala* 'dominated by bile', or *śleṣmala* 'dominated by phlegm'. All three are permanent parts of the human body (Sūtra-sthāna 18.48):

nityāḥ prāṇa-bhṛtāṃ dehe vāta-pitta-kaphās trayaḥ
vikṛtāḥ prakṛti-sthā vā tān bubhutseta paṇḍitaḥ

Wind, bile, phlegm — these three are always present in
the body of creatures. A physician should try to find out
whether they are in their natural state or transformed.

The distinction between natural and transformed states is important, as Sūtra-sthāna 20.9 explains:

sarva-śarīra-carās tu vāta-pitta-śleṣmānaḥ, sarvasmiñ charīre kupitâkupitāḥ śubhâśubhāni kurvanti; prakṛti-bhūtāḥ śubhāny upacaya-bala-varṇa-prasādâdīni, aśu-bhāni punar vikṛtim āpannā vikāra-saṃjñakāni.

Wind, bile, and phlegm, in fact, move throughout the whole body and bring about in the whole body good and bad results according as they are riled or not; in their natural state [they bring about] good results like growth, strength, [good] complexion, happiness, etc., but when they have undergone acts of transformation, [they bring about] bad results, i.e., what are called transformations (viz., illnesses).

Wind, bile, and phlegm are also listed among the waste products of the body in Sūtra-sthāna 28.4:

tatrâhāra-prasādâkhyo rasaḥ kiṭṭaṃca malâkhyam abhinirvartate. kiṭṭāt sveda-mūtra-purīṣa-vāta-pitta-śleṣmāṇaḥ karṇâkṣi-nāsikâsya-loma-kūpa-prajanana-malāḥ keśa-śmaśru-loma-nakhâdayaś câvayavāḥ puṣyanti. puṣyanti tu āhāra-rasād rasa-rudhira-māṃsa-medo'sthi-majja-śukraûjāṃsi

When this [food is digested], chyle, also known as food essence and refuse, called waste, evolve. From the refuse prosper sweat, urine, faeces, wind, bile, phlegm, excreta of the ear, eye, nose, mouth, hair follicles, and the sex organs, as well as the [body] parts: hair of the head, beard, body hair, nails, etc. From the food essence prosper chyle, blood, flesh, bones, marrow, semen, vital strength

The inclusion of the human waste products, presumably those not yet expelled, among the parts of the body (cf., the Buddhist lists) may surprise us, but it has its parallel in the Indian theory of the state that included the ally and sometimes even the enemy among the constituents of a polity.[68] The whole functioning unit is visualised. A small output of faeces and urine is not described as the consequence of a medical problem but as a symptom, if not a cause, of it in Sūtra-sthāna 17.70f.

kṣīṇe śakṛti cântrāṇi pīḍayann iva mārutaḥ
rūkṣasyônnamayan kukṣiṃ tiryag ūrdhvaṃ ca gacchati

mūtra-kṣaye mūtra-kṛcchraṃ mūtra-vaivarṇyam eva ca
pipāsā bādhate câsya mukhaṃ ca pariśuṣyati

And if the stool is diminished, wind squeezes, as it were, the intestines; lifting the abdomen of the dehydrated [person], the wind goes sideways and upwards. If urine is diminished, dysurea and discoloration of the urine [is found], and thirst afflicts [a person], and his mouth gets dry.

Wind, bile, and phlegm can become riled and, in consequence, cause illness. The primary cause for this is faulty nutrition, as Sūtra-sthāna 18.7 spells out:

ayaṃ tv atra viśeṣaḥ: śīta-rūkṣa-laghu-viśada-śramōpa-vāsâtikarśaṇa-kṣapaṇâdibhir vāyuḥ prakupitas tvaṅ-māṃsa-śoṇitâdīny abhibhūya śophaṃ janayati; sa kṣiprôtthāna-praśamo bhavati . . . , uṣṇa-tīkṣṇa-kaṭuka-kṣāra-lavaṇâmlâjīrṇa-bhojanair agny-ātapa-pratāpaiś ca pittaṃ prakupitaṃ tvaṅ-māṃsa-śoṇitâdīny abhibhūya śōthaṃ janayati; sa kṣiprôtthāna-praśamo bhavati . . . guru-madhura-śīta-snigdhair atisvapnâvyāyāmâdibhiś ca śleṣmā prakupitas tvaṅ-māṃsa-śoṇitâdīny abhibhūya śothaṃ janayati; sa kṛcchrôtthāna-praśamobhavati

There is this difference: Riled by [the intake of] cold, non-unctuous, light, non-slimy [food], by exertion, fasting, excessive emaciation and elimination, wind afflicts the skin, flesh, blood, etc., and causes swelling; this [swelling] appears and calms down quickly . . . Riled by [the intake of] hot, pungent, bitter, alkaline, saline, sour, and heavy food and by [exposure to] the heat of fire or the sun, bile afflicts the skin, flesh, blood, etc., and causes swelling; this [swelling] appears and calms down quickly . . . Riled by [the intake of] heavy, sweet, cold, and unctuous [food], by excessive sleep, lack of exercise, etc., phlegm afflicts the skin, flesh, blood, etc., and causes swelling; this [swelling] takes a long time to appear and to calm down (i.e., to be cured)

Besides food, the seasons are a major factor that can rile wind, bile, and phlegm. Sūtra-sthāna 6.33f. says:

ādāna-durbale dehe paktā bhavati durbalaḥ
sa varṣāsv anilādīnāṃ dūcaṇair bādhyate punaḥ
bhū-bāṣpān megha-nisyandāt pākād amlāj jalasya ca
varṣāsv agni-bale kṣīṇe kupyanti pavanâdayaḥ

In the body, weakened by dehydration (during summer), the power of digestion is [also] weakened; during the rains (which follow summer) [the power of digestion] is further afflicted by the vitiations of wind, etc. When the power of digestion during the rains is reduced due to vapors coming from the soil, rainfall, and increase of acidity in water, wind, etc., become riled.

varṣā-śītôcitâṅgānāṃ sahasaîvārka-raśmibhiḥ
taptānām ācitaṃ pittaṃ prāyaḥ śaradi kupyati (Sū 6.41)

When the limbs that are used to rain and cold are suddenly heated by the rays of the sun, the accumulated bile usually becomes riled in the fall.[69]

caya-prakopa-praśamāḥ pittâdīnāṃ yathākramam
bhavanty ekaikaśaḥ ṣaṭsu kāleṣv abhrâgamâdiṣu
gatiḥ kāla-kṛtā caîṣā cayâdyā punar ucyate (Sū 17.114f.)

Accumulation, anger, and calming of bile, etc., happen in due order one by one in the seasons beginning with the monsoon, and this process, i.e., accumulation, etc., is said to be caused by the seasons.

But such aggravation of the bile can also be the consequence of bad treatment (Sū 14.14): *pitta-prakopo, mūrcchā . . . atisvinnasya lakṣaṇam* ('anger of the bile, fainting . . . are the sign of over-fomentation'). Due to various activities, from the suppression of natural urges to practices incompatible with the location or season, 'wind, etc., become riled, and the blood in the head vitiated; hence illnesses with various symptoms arise in the head' (Sū 17.11).[70] By excessive acts, from loud speech to long walks and emaciation, 'the increased wind enters the vessels in the head and gets riled;[71] then a sharp pain arises in (the head) from the wind' (Sū 17.18).[72] 'By (the consumption of food having) acrid, sour, or saline (taste), alkalies and alcohols, by anger, by (exposure to) sun and fire, the bile in the head becomes vitiated and causes illness in the head' (Sū 17.22).[73] 'By the comforts of sitting, the comforts of sleep, excessive consumption of heavy and unctuous (food), the phlegm in the head becomes vitiated and causes illness in the head' (Sū 17.24).[74]

The symptoms differ, depending on which of the three causes is involved. All three causes may be involved at the same time, and the sum of the symptoms can be attributed to the power of each of these causes: 'Because of wind there is pain, giddiness, shaking of the head; because of bile there is a burning sensation, intoxication (and) thirst; because of phlegm there is heaviness and drowsiness (all this together) in an illness of the head born from (all) three faults' (Sū 17.26):

vātāc chūlaṃ bhramaḥ kampaḥ, pittād dāho madas tṛṣā
kaphād gurutvaṃ tandrā ca śiro-roge tri-doṣa-je

In this last stanza the symptoms caused by the wind, bile, and phlegm alone are repeated in abbreviated form, as they occur jointly when all three causes are involved. Wind, bile, and phlegm — riled and causes for an illness — are here referred to as 'the three faults'.

Diseases are generally cured by attacking the underlying cause. '(Medicines that are) sweet, sour, and salty defeat wind; (those that are) astringent, sweet, and bitter (defeat) bile; (those that are) astringent, pungent, and bitter (defeat) phlegm' (Sū 1.66):

svādv-amla-lavaṇa vāyuṃ kaṣāya-svādu-tiktakāḥ
jayanti pittaṃ, śleṣmāṇaṃ kaṣāya-kamu-tiktakāḥ

A certain medicated enema is called 'wind-killing' (Sū 7.19 *vāta-ghnam* cf., 24 *vāta-ghnyas* and 13.15 *māruta-ghnam*); 'sweet taste . . . kills bile, poison, and wind' (Sū 26.43/1 *tatra madhuro rasaḥ. . . pitta-viṣa-māruta-ghnas*); 'for these fats are prescribed as knocking off wind, bile, and phlegm' (Sū 1.88 *snehā hy ete ca vihitā vāta-pitta-kaphâpahāḥ*); 'ghee removes bile and wind' (Sū 13.14 *ghṛtaṃ pittānila-haraṃ*). Such strong expressions are also found in sentences where wind, bile, and phlegm as targets of medication are parallel to diseases: a certain concoction 'knocks off cough, hiccup, dyspnoea, and phlegm' (Sū 2.27 *kāsa-hikkā-śvāsa-kaphāpahā*), 'bamboo seed . . . kills phlegm and bile and kills fat, worms, and poison' (Sū 27.20 *kapha-pitta-hā medaḥ-krimi-viṣa-ghnaś ca . . . veṇu-yavo mataḥ*). Among other benefits, 'destruction of faults and increase of the digestive power is born from physical exercise' (Sū 7.32 *dośa-kṣayo'gni-vṛddhiś ca vyāyāmād upajāyate*).

The direct contrast to the 'riling' of wind, bile, and phlegm is their 'calming down'. '(Urine) when drunk, calms bile' (Sū 1.98 *śleṣmāṇaṃ śamayet pītaṃ*) 'and the wind is calmed' (when oil is massaged into the feet) (Sū 5.91 *mārutaś côpaśāmyati*); note also the passage quoted earlier from Sūtra-sthāna 18.7: *vāyuḥ prakupitas . . . kṣiprōtthāna-praśamo bhavati*, where *prakupita* and *praśama* contrast.[75] When all three, wind, bile, and phlegm, were riled and cause illness, they are referred to as the three faults: 'The black-bucks (i.e., their meat) . . . calm the three faults' (Sū 27.77 *tri-doṣa-śamanāḥ*). 'Killing the three faults' (*tri-doṣa-ghnam*)[76] and 'calming the three faults' (*tri-doṣa-śamanī*) are used as parallel expressions in Sū 27.89. Combatting 'faults' can be expressed as 'killing' them, e.g., Sūtra-sthāna 1.100f. where 'goat's (urine) strikes down faults; a cow's (urine) is fault-killing' (*ājaṃ . . . doṣān nihanti; . . . gavyaṃ . . . doṣa-ghnaṃ*). A stanza, apparently quoted from another source, stresses the importance of removing a fault altogether (Sū 26.85):

> *bhavanti câtra ślokāḥ:*
> *yat kiñcid doṣam āsrāvya na nirharati kāyataḥ*
> *āhāra-jātaṃ tat sarvam ahitāyôpapadyate*
>
> And there are stanzas:
> All drugs and diets that liquefy a certain fault but do not
> remove it from the body are ultimately unwholesome.

Cakrapāṇi's commentary suggests that this total removal is achieved through emetics and purgatives; this interpretation is consistent with the teaching of Sūtra-sthāna 16.20:

> *doṣāḥ kadācit kupyanti jitā laṅgana-pācanaiḥ*
> *jitāḥ saṃśodhanair ye tu na teṣāṃ punar-udbhavaḥ*
>
> Sometimes faults that are defeated by fasting and digestive
> drugs are riled [again]; but those that are defeated
> by elimination therapies do not recur.

A disease is easy to cure (*sukha-sādhya*) if the fault (*doṣa*) is of a different quality than the affected constituent of the body or if there is only one fault (*doṣaś caîkaḥ*).[77] A disease is difficult to cure (*kṛcchra-sādhya*) or merely palliable (*yāpya*) if it is caused by two faults (*dvidoṣa-jam*; 16f.), but one should refuse (*pratyākhyeya*) treatment for a disease caused by three faults (*tri-doṣa-ja*;19).[78] It may be for metrical reasons that here the terms *saṃsarga* and *saṃnipāta* for the combination of two and three faults are not used; they do occur in Sūtra-sthāna 17.41f.[79] and are defined in Vimāna-sthāna 6.11.

At this time we should take a closer look at how *doṣa* 'fault' is used in relation to wind, bile, and phlegm. 'Wind, not riled . . . dries up the faults . . . ; but riled in the body it afflicts the body with various types of transformation (i.e., diseases)' (Sū 12.8: *vāyur . . . doṣa-saṃśoṣaṇḥ . . . bhavaty akupitaḥ; kupitas tu khalu śarīre śarīraṃ nānāvidhair vikārair upatapati*); this implies that wind which is not riled is not itself a fault (*doṣa*). This fact can explain the contrast of *doṣa* and *dhātu* in Sūtra-sthāna 1.67:

> *kiṃcid doṣa-praśamanaṃ kiṃcid dhātu-pradūṣaṇam*
> *svastha-vṛttau mataṃ kiṃcit tri-vidhaṃ dravyam ucyate*
>
> Medication is said to be of three kinds: some calms down faults, some vitiates elements, some is meant for maintenance of positive health.

Here it is the fault that must be calmed down, whereas an element can be vitiated (until it becomes a fault).[80] It is therefore not legitimate (as far as Caraka and other old medical texts are concerned) to introduce the notion of 'fault' in a discussion of the healthy body, as is often done in modem translations. I shall give one example of this practice. Sūtra-sthāna 5.4 *yāvad dhy asyâśanam aśitam anupahatya prakṛtiṃ . . . jarāṃ gacchati* should be translated as: 'The amount of food which, without upsetting the physique, gets digested'. Cakrapāṇi's commentary explains the word 'physique' of the text with 'equilibrium of wind, etc., and chyle, etc.' (*prakṛtim vātâdīnāṃ rasâdīnāṃ ca sāmyâvasthām*). This gloss, which seems unobjectionable, is incorrectly reflected in the modern translation of the Caraka-saṃhitā by R. K. Sharma and Bh. Dash as 'without disturbing the equilibrium (of *dhātus* and *doṣas* of the body)'.[81] Since wind, etc., are not yet disturbed, they are not 'faults'. A modern Siddha author[82] still preserves the old distinction. He writes: 'When these *thridhatus* become abnormal or when their mutual harmony is disturbed (in which role they are called *thridosha*) they bring about ill health'.[83]

'Wind, bile, and phlegm when spoiled become spoilers of all these,[84] because that is the nature of a fault' (*teṣāṃ sarveṣām eva vāta-pitta-śleṣmāṇo duṣṭā dūṣayitāro bhavanti, doṣa-svabhāvāt* Śā 6.18). A contrast develops between wind, bile, and phlegm that have become faults (*doṣa*)—and hence spoilers — and the elements of the body (*dhātu*) that are going to be spoiled (*dūṣya*). Thus, we read in Ci 6.8:

kaphaḥ sa-pittaḥ pavanaś ca doṣā
medo 'sra-śukrāmbu-vasā-lasīkāḥ
majjā rasaûjaḥ piśitaṃ ca dūṣyāḥ
pramehiṇām, viṃśatir eva mehāḥ

Phlegm with bile, and wind, are the faults; and fat, blood,
semen, water, lymph, marrow, chyle, vitality, and flesh
are the [elements] to be spoiled [in the bodies] of diabetics;
there are twenty [kinds of] diabetes.

And in Ci 21.15 we read about the skin disease *visarpa*:

raktaṃ lasīkā tvaṅ māṃsaṃ dūṣyaṃ doṣās trayo malāḥ
visarpāṇāṃ samutpattau vijñeyāḥ sapta dhātavaḥ

Blood, lymph, skin, flesh are what is to be spoiled, the
three faults are the impurities; seven elements should be
recognized in the origin of *visarpa*.

Here the three faults seem to be included together with the four named elements (*dhātu*) to bring the number of *dhātus* up to seven. A strict equation *dhātu* = *dūṣya*, however, is only found in later texts (*Aṣṭāṅga-saṃgraha* and *Aṣṭāṅga-hṛdaya-saṃhitā*; see later in the chapter).

The worldview of the Sāṃkhya philosophy, including its ontology of the three 'strands' (*guṇa*), dominates the general thinking in the *Caraka-saṃhitā*, even though notions current in other philosophical schools are also used wherever convenient. Sūtra-sthāna 1.57f. displays key terms of Sāṃkhya:

vāyuḥ pittaṃ kaphaś cōktaḥ śārīro doṣa-saṃgrahaḥ
mānasaḥ punar uddiṣṭo rajaś ca tama eva ca
praśāmyaty auṣadhaiḥ pūrvo daiva-yukti-vyapāśrayaiḥ
mānaso jñāna-vijñāna-dhairya-smṛti-samādhibhiḥ

Wind, bile, phlegm are called the corporeal sum of faults;
the mental [sum of faults] again is taught as *rajas* and
tamas.[85] The former [sum of faults] is calmed down by
therapies relying on divine intervention and rational remedies;
the mental [sum of faults is calmed down] by knowledge,
insight, steadfastness, memory, and meditation.

These notions are expanded in Vimāna-sthāna 6.5:

rajas tamaś ca mānasau doṣau; tayor vikārāḥ kāma-krodha-lobha-mohêrṣyā-māna-mada-śoka-cintôdvega-bhaya-harṣādayaḥ. vāta-pitta-śleṣmāṇas tu khalu śārīrā doṣāḥ; teṣām api ca vikārā jvarâtīsāra-śopha-śoṣa-śvāsa-meha-kuṣṭhâdayaḥ

rajas and *tamas* are the mental faults; their transformations are desire, wrath, greed, delusion, envy, conceit, intoxication, grief, mental excitement, fear, arousal, etc. Wind, bile, and phlegm, however, are corporeal faults; and their transformations are fever, diarrhea, swelling, dryness, dyspnoea, urinary disorders, skin diseases, etc.

The attempt to link the three faults of medical theory[86] and the strands of Sāṃkhya[87] remains superficial: the numbers do not match, since the three faults are paired with only two of the three strands. While it is doubtful that *rajas* and *tamas* were called 'faults' in classical Sāṃkhya texts, preclassical texts like *Mahābhārata* XII.212.25–31 do contrast the 'good' *sattva* with the comparatively 'bad' *rajas* and *tamas*.

sāttviko rājasaś caîva tāmasaś caîva te trayaḥ
tri-vidhā vedanā yeṣu prasūtā sarva-sādhanā | 25 |
praharcaḥ prītir ānandaḥ sukhaṃ saṃśānta-cittatā
akutaścit kutaścid vā cittataḥ sāttviko guṇaḥ | 26 |
atuṣṭiḥ paritāpaś ca śoko lobhas tathâkṣamā
liṅgāni rajasas tāni dṛśyante hetv-ahetutaḥ | 27 |
avivekas tathā mohaḥ pramādaḥ svapna-tandritā
kathaṃcid api vartante vividhās tāmasā guṇāḥ | 28 |
tatra yat prīti-saṃyuktaṃ kāye manasi vā bhavet

vartate sāttviko bhāva ity apekṣeta tat tathā | 29 |
yat tu saṃtāpa-saṃyuktamaprītikaram ātmanaḥ
pravṛttaṃ raja ity eva tatas tad abhicintayet | 30 |
atha yan moha-saṃyuktaṃ kāye manasi vā bhavet
apratarkyam avijñeyaṃ tamas tad upadhārayet | 31 |

[the state] based on *sattva*, the one based on *rajas*, and the one based on *tamas*, these three, in which threefold feeling is born that effects everything. Thrill, love, pleasure, happiness, peace of mind, . . . is the quality based on *sattva*. Dissatisfaction, anguish, sadness, greed, and impatience, these are perceived as the signs of *rajas*, whether caused [by it] or not. Lack of distinction and delusion, carelessness, sluggishness of sleep, somehow are the various qualities of *tamas*. This being so, what there is in body or mind that is joined with love, that is based on *sattva*; thus one should see it. What the Self has that is joined with anguish [and] creates displeasure, that is *rajas* in action; thus one should hence consider it. But what is joined with delusion in body or mind, can not be figured out [and] can not be known, that one should consider *tamas*.[88]

Caraka espouses similar views in Śā 1.36:

rajas-tamobhyāṃ yuktasya saṃyogo'yam anantavān
tābhāṃ nirākṛtābhyāṃ tu sattva-vṛddhyā nivartate

This connection [with the senses and their objects] is unending for one who is linked with *rajas* and *tamas*; with these two done away, it ceases through the growth of *sattva*.

And Śā 1.142: mokṣo *rajas-tamo* 'bhāvāt 'Liberation [derives] from the absence of *rajas* and *tamas*'.[89] *Sattva* is placed on a different level from *rajas* and *tamas* also in Śā 4.34–36:

tatra trayaḥś arīra-doṣā vāta-pitta-śleṣmāṇaḥ, te śarīraṃ dūṣayanti; dvau punaḥ sattva-doṣau rajas tamaś ca, tau sattvaṃ dūṣayataḥ. tābhyāṃ ca sattva-śarīrābhyāṃ duṣ-mābhyāṃ vikṛtir upajāyate, nôpajâyate câpraduṣṭābhyām. tatraś arīraṃ yoni-viśeṣāc caturvidham uktam agre. tri-vidhaṃ khalu sattvaṃ śuddhaṃ, rājasaṃ, tāmasam iti

There are three faults of the body [i.e.] wind, bile, phlegm, they spoil the body; then there are two faults of the *sattva* 'mind'[90] [i.e.] *rajas* and *tamas*, they spoil *sattva* 'mind'. With these two [i.e.] *sattva* and body spoiled, a deviating transformation occurs, and it does not occur when they are not spoiled. Now, the body has been said at the beginning to be of four kinds due to different origins.[91] The *sattva* is of three kinds: pure, admixed with *rajas*, ad mixed with *tamas*

It will be necessary to examine a few other occurrences of the term *doṣa* in the *Caraka-saṃhitā*, where it has been taken to denote 'humor'. The stanzas Sūtrasthāna 17.41–62 go through the various combinations, where one, two, or all three of the causal elements, i.e., wind, bile, and phlegm, have grown in excess to various degrees or are diminished; there are further combinations where one or two of them are grown in excess, while the remainder is diminished. In this context the word *doṣa* 'fault' is used twice:

yathā vṛddhais tathā kṣīṇair doṣaiḥ syuḥ pañcaviṃśatiḥ
vṛddhi-kṣaya-kṛtaś cânyo vikalpa upadekṣyate |43|

As there are with the increased [faults], thus there would also be twenty-five [combinations] with the diminished faults; and the other condition [of twelve more combinations] will be taught as effected by growth and diminution.

doṣāḥ pravṛddhāḥ svaṃ liṅgaṃ darśayanti yathābalam
kṣīṇa jahati liṅgaṃ svaṃ samāḥ svaṃ karma kurvate |62|

The much increased faults show their mark in accordance with their strength; those that are diminished abandon their mark, those that are even, do their proper work.

A strict interpretation might suggest that here wind, bile, and phlegm, even in their normal and healthy state, are called faults. But one should also notice that the expression *doṣa* is used in immediate proximity to *kṣīṇa* and *pravṛddha*, terms that indicate pathological deviation, i.e., a fault. In the intervening stanzas all references are to *vāta* / *māruta* / *vāyu* / *anila* / *samīraṇa*, *pitta*, and *kapha* / *śleṣman*, not to *doṣa*.[92]

The prose sentences Sūtra-sthāna 12.8–12 attempt to place wind, bile, and phlegm in a correspondence of the microcosmos versus macrocosmos, possibly in a reprise of ideas found in the upaniṣads. In the beginning, wind is described as a constituent of the body, first in its natural state, i.e., non-riled (*akupita*), then riled (*kupita*); subsequently, it is detailed as a force in the outside world (*loke*), first in its natural state involving the kindling of fire, the showering of rains, etc., then in its riled form involving the uprooting of trees, causing earthquakes, etc. Finally, Lord Wind (Vāyu) is the eternal cause of the universe; he is Lord Viṣṇu. 'It is Agni (the god of fire) alone, represented by bile in the body, which brings about good or bad effects according to its being non-riled or riled, i.e., digestion or indigestion' (Sū 12.11 *agnir eva śarīre pittântargataḥ kupitâkupitaḥ śubhâśubhāni karoti tad yathā paktim apaktiṃ*). Similarly Soma, the moon as the receptacle of water, is represented in the body by phlegm.

The dominant position of wind is also evident in Sūtrasthāna 17.115–18. In the preceding stanzas, 112f., we read about the threefold way of faults (*doṣa*): they may be diminished, stay as they are, or they may grow. It is not certain that the word *doṣa* continues in the following stanzas:

gatiś ca dvi-vidhā dṛṣṭā prākṛtī vaikṛtī ca yā | 115 |
pittād evōṣmaṇaḥ paktir narāṇām upajāyate
tac ca pittaṃ prakupitaṃ vikārān kurute bahūn | 116 |
prākṛtas tu balaṃ śleṣmā vikṛto mala ucyate
sa caīvaûjaḥ smṛtaḥ kāye sa ca pāpmōpadiśyate | 117 |
sarvā hi ceṣṭā vātena sa prāṇaḥ prāṇināṃ smṛtaḥ
tenaîva rogā jāyante tena caīvôparudhyate | 118 |

And there is a twofold way, viz., natural and transformed.
From bile is born men's digestive force of heat;
and that bile, if riled, effects many transformations (i.e.,
illnesses). Natural phlegm is called "strength," transformed
[phlegm is called] "refuse": the one is remembered
as vital force[93] in the body, the other is taught to
be evil. All movement, indeed, is [caused] by wind;
[wind] is remembered as the vital breath of living
beings; by the very same [wind, if riled], diseases are
born, and by it one is led to one's death.

If *doṣa* is understood in these stanzas as a referent, this should strictly only apply to the 'transformed way' (*vaikṛtī gatiḥ*), when wind, bile, and phlegm have become 'faults', not the natural way when they carry on with their beneficial functions.

Two passages will clarify the relation of wind, bile, and phlegm with the body elements (*dhātu*). Sūtra-sthāna 17.63:

vātâtdīnāṃ rasâdīnāṃ malānām ojasas tathā
kṣayās tatrânilâdīnām uktaṃ saṃkṣīṇa-lakṣaṇam

Diminuitions occur of wind, etc., chyle, etc., waste products
and vitality. Regarding this, the characteristics of
diminuition of wind, etc., have [already] been told.

In the following stanzas the diminuition of chyle, blood, flesh, fat, bone, marrow, semen, i.e., the elements (*dhātu*), and of faeces, urine and 'other waste products' are described. It is clear, therefore, that wind, etc., were not counted among the chyle, etc., i.e., the elements (*dhātu*). Sūtra-sthāna 19.5 deals with the relation of wind etc., and the elements.

> *sarva eva nijā vikārā nânyatra vāta-pitta-kaphebhyo nirvartante, yathā hi śakuniḥ sarvaṃ divasam api paripatan svāṃ chāyāṃ nâtivartate, tathā sva-dhātu-vaiṣamya-nimittāḥ sarve vikārā vāta-pitta-kaphān nâtivartante. vāta-pitta-śleṣmaṇāṃ punaḥ sthāna-saṃsthāna-prakṛti-viśeṣān abhisamīkṣya tad-ātmakān api ca sarva-vikārāṃs tān evôpadiśanti buddhimantaḥ.*

> All the endogenous diseases occur only [in connection] with wind, bile, or phlegm; for as a bird cannot transgress its own shadow even though flying throughout the day, so also all endogenous diseases caused by an imbalance of one's body elements cannot transgress wind, bile, and phlegm. Again, considering the specific location, symptoms and causes of wind, bile, and phlegm, the wise teach all these transformations (i.e., diseases) as having that (i.e., wind, bile, or phlegm) as their identity.[94]

To sum up: the older parts of the *Caraka-saṃhitā* consider wind, bile, and phlegm in their natural state as elements (*dhātu*) and only in their riled condition as faults (*doṣa*). Health is the balance of the elements (*dhātu*).[95] The three faults (*doṣa*) are put in an awkward relation with the two less valuable strands/qualities (*guṇa*).

The *Suśruta-samhitā*

I shall first present the evidence found in the Sūtra-sthāna. The presentation of Āyurvedic theory is strikingly different from that in the *Caraka-saṃhitā*, but some peculiarities of Suśruta's teaching — I would call them innovations[96] — have received little attention so far. The reasons for this shall be discussed later. The three faults (*doṣa*) are always part of the human body. Sūtra-sthāna 15.3:

> *doṣa-dhātu-mala-mūlaṃ hi śarīraṃ*

> For the body is rooted in faults, elements, and waste products.

Sūtra-sthāna 15.37–41:

vailakṣaṇyāc charīrāṇām asthāyitvāt tathaîva ca
doṣa-dhātu-malānāṃ tu parimāṇaṃ na vidyate |37|
eṣāṃ samatvaṃ yac câpi bhiṣagbhir avadhāryate
na tat svāsthyād ṛte śakyaṃ vaktum anyena hetunā |38|
doṣâdīnāṃ tv asamatām anumānena lakṣayet
aprasannêndriyaṃ vikṣya puruṣaṃ kuśalo bhiṣak |39|
svasthasya rakṣaṇaṃ kuryād asvasthasya tu buddhimān
kṣapayed bṛṃhayec câpi doṣa-dhātu-malān bhiṣak
tāvad yāvad arogaḥ syād etad sāmyasya lakṣaṇam |40|
sama-doṣaḥ samâgniś ca sama-dhātu-mala-kriyaḥ
prasannâctmêndriya-manāḥ svastha ity abhidhīyate |41|

Because the bodies vary [from one person to another] and because they are not static, an exact measure of the faults, elements, and waste products is not known. And their balance that is ascertained by physicians cannot be told by any other reason except on the grounds of perfect health. But a skilled physician would by inference characterize an imbalance of the faults, etc., when he observes a man whose faculties are unsettled. The physician shall protect the healthy [man], but shall weaken and strengthen [as the case demands] faults, elements, and waste products of an unhealthy one, until he is healthy; that is the mark of balance. A person with balanced faults, balanced digestive fire, balanced actions of the elements and the waste products, whose self, senses, and mind are settled, is called healthy.

Sūtra-sthāna 21.7 lists the organs where wind, bile, and phlegm are primarily located; it concludes: *etāni khalu doṣānāṃ sthānāny avyāpannānām* 'These are the locations of the faults when they are not afflicted'.

The role of wind, bile, and phlegm is comparable to that in the treatises discussed earlier, but is more powerful and exclusive. Sūtra-sthāna 21.3 tells us:

vāta-pitta-śleṣmāṇa eva deha-saṃbhava-hetavaḥ. tair evâvyāpannair adho-madhyôrdhva-saṃniviṣṭaiḥ śarīram idaṃ dhāryate 'gāram iva sthūṇābhis tisṛbhir, ataś ca tri-sthūṇam āhur eke. ta eva ca vyāpannāḥ pralaya-hetavaḥ. tad ebhir eva śoṇita-caturthaiḥ saṃbhava-sthiti-pra-layeṣv apy avirahitaṃ śarīraṃ bhavati.

> Wind, bile, and phlegm[97] alone are the causes for the constitution of the body. By them alone, if they are unimpaired, occupying [respectively] the lower, middle, and upper [parts of the body] is this body held up like a house with three supporting poles; hence some call [the body] "three-pillared."[98]Impaired, these same are the cause of dissolution. This body is not separated from these same [three], with blood as the fourth, in its origin, stay, and dissolution.

Certain medicinal plasters remove swelling caused by wind, by bile, by phlegm, and by a combination of all three of them (Su 37.3–7: *pralepo vāta-śopha-hṛt;... pralepaḥ pitta-śopha-hṛt;... pralepaḥśleṣma-śopha-jit ... lepo'yam sānnipātika-śopha-hṛt*). 'Wind, bile, and phlegm alone are the root of all diseases' (Sū 24.8: *sarve-ṣāṃ ca vyādhīnāṃ vāta-pitta-śleṣ māṇa eva mūlam*). Blood sometimes joins the other three causes as a fourth, as in Sūtra-sthāna 1.24: *śārīrās tv anna-pāna-mūlā vāta-pitta-kapha-śoṇita-sannipāta-vaiṣamya-nimittāḥ* 'But bodily (diseases), rooted in food and drink are caused by an imbalance of wind, bile, phlegm, blood,[99] or their combination'. Imbalance (*vaiṣamya*) of wind, bile, and phlegm as the cause of illness was not found in the texts studied earlier; the closest is the statement of *Caraka*, Sūtra-sthāna, 7.39 that people with balanced (*sama*) congenital wind, bile, and phlegm have the best constitution. We read in Suśruta's work of the riling (*prakopa*) and calming (*praśama*) of the faults (Sū 1.34f.). Sūtra-sthāna 15.36 describes the impact of a riled fault:

> *doṣaḥ prakupito dhātūn kṣapayaty ātma-tejasā*
> *iddhaḥ sva-tejasā vahnir ukhā-gatam ivôdakam*

> A riled fault destroys the bodily elements by its own glare, as a kindled fire [evaporates] water in a pot with its own flame.

Therefore, a fault must be calmed down (Sū 18.7):

> *avidagdheṣu śopheṣu hitam ālepanaṃ bhavet*
> *yathāsvaṃ doṣa-śamanaṃ dāha-kaṇḍū-rujâpaham*

> A medical plaster of the alepana class would prove beneficial in swellings that suppurated, inasmuch as it

calms the faults [and] pushes off (= removes) burning,
itching, and pain [the typical consequences of bile,
phlegm, and wind].

Since the balance of faults, bodily elements, and excreta is essential for a person's well-being, any diminution of these must be countered and corrected. Sūtra-sthāna 15.29:

doṣa-dhātu-mala-kṣīṇo bala-kṣīṇo'pi vā naraḥ
sva-yoni-vardhanaṃ yat tad anna-pānaṃ prakāṅkṣati

A man deficient in faults, bodily elements, and excreta,[100]
and deficient in strength desires food and drink
that will strengthen their respective procreation.

This desire of the patient is not a morbid wish to be discouraged but considered medically proper in Suśruta's Cikitsita-sthāna 33.3f:

doṣāḥ kṣīṇā bṛṃhayitavyāḥ, kupitāḥ praśamayitavyāḥ,
vṛddhā nirhartavyāḥ, samāḥ paripālyā iti siddhāntaḥ. prā-
dhānyena vamana-virecane vartete nirharaGe doṣāṇām.

Diminished faults must be strengthened, riled [faults]
calmed, increased [faults] removed, balanced [faults] protected:
that is the authoritative doctrine. Most prominently,
emetics and purgatives are used to remove the faults.

This intentional strengthening of the 'faults' (*doṣa*) is a new element in Suśruta's work; all previously discussed works sought only to calm or remove and destroy the faults. Such expressions are even still found in the *Suśruta-saṃhitā*. In Sūtra-sthāna 11.3 we read that 'alkali is most important . . . because it kills the three faults' (*kṣāraḥ pradhānatamaḥ . . . tri-doṣa-ghnatvād*); 'rainwater kills the three faults' (Sū 45.26 *gaga-nâmbu tri-doṣa-ghnaṃ*), and among the benefits of a medicinal plaster called *ālepana* or *kalka*, applied to an ulcer, is *anantardoṣatā* 'absence of faults inside' (Sū 18.6). In Sūtra-sthāna 45 (*madhu-vargaḥ*), v. 141 we learn that:

doṣa-traya-haraṃ pakvam, āmam amlaṃ tri-doṣa-kṛt

Mature [honey] removes the three faults, raw [and] sour
[honey] creates the three faults.

What could have caused a development such that the balance of the faults becomes an ideal to be preserved and that diminished faults must be increased? Or the notion that the three faults are an essential, even beneficial, part in the make-up of the human body? Actually, Suśruta is quite explicit about his thoughts on this subject. He says in Sūtra-sthāna 24.8:

> *sarveṣāṃ ca vyādhīnāṃ vāta-pitta-śleṣmāṇa eva mūlaṃ; tal-liṅgatvād dṛṣṭa-phalatvād āgamāc ca. yathā hi kṛtsnaṃ vikāra-jātaṃ viśva-rūpeṇâvasthitaṃ sattva-rajas-tamāṃsi na vyatiricyante, evam eva kṛtsnaṃ vikāra-jātam viśva-rūpeṇāvasthitam avyatiricya vāta-pitta-śleṣmāṇo vartante. doṣa-dhātu-mala-saṃsargād āyatana-viśeṣān nimittataś caîṣāṃ vikalpaḥ. doṣa-dūṣiteṣv atyarthaṃ dhātuṣu saṃjñā: rasa-jo'yaṃ, śoṇita-jo 'yaṃ, māṃsa-jo 'yaṃ, medo-jo 'yam, asthi-jo 'yaṃ, majja-jo 'yaṃ, śukra-jo 'yaṃ vyādhir iti.*

> Wind, bile, and phlegm alone are the root of all diseases, because [the diseases] carry their distinguishing mark, because the fruit [of wind, bile, and phlegm] is seen, and because the tradition [says so]. For as [the three strands] *sattva*, *rajas*, and *tamas* are not separate from the universe, [which is] nothing but a transformation [of the three strands], [and] established with all phenomenal appearances; thus wind, bile, and phlegm exist without being separate from everything that is a transformation (i.e., illness) [and are] established with all phenomenal appearances. Because of the contact of faults, bodily elements, and waste products, because of the difference of locations, and because of their causation, there are different forms [of disease]. As bodily elements are exceedingly aggravated by the faults, a term [viz., a technical expression, as in the following] is created: "this illness is born from chyle, this from blood, this from flesh, this from fat, this from bone, this from marrow, this from semen."

There is no doubt that the Sāṃkhya philosophy played a major role in the medical texts; the five elements with their qualities are important notions in the medical man's view of the body and the world. The discovery of a homology between the strands (*guṇa*) that make up the physical world and the three faults (*doṣa*) that move and eventually destroy the body must have been overwhelming, especially when we consider that the word *guṇa* had expanded from its earlier meaning of three strands in a braid — or the strands of the physical world — to the meaning of 'quality, good quality, virtue', the antonym of *doṣa*, 'fault'. This homology is superior to Caraka's clumsy attempt to link the two systems: *rajas* and *tamas* (the somewhat 'inferior' *guṇas*) leading to mental illness, on the one hand; wind, bile, and phlegm as the three faults causing corporeal illness, on the other. In Suśruta's view the correspondence is symmetrical: just as the three strands of Sāṃkhya transform themselves into the world through the subtle and gross elements (*tan-mātra*, *bhūta*), the three faults cause illnesses through the bodily elements (*dhātu*). This is the main intellectual achievement of Suśruta, which has had a lasting effect on later authors.[101]

The author of the Uttara-tantra ('Supplementary Chapter'), apparently a later addition to the main text of the Suśruta-saṃhitā,[102] is commonly dubbed Suśruta the Younger or Suśruta II. In Uttara-tantra 66.9 he seems to identify the three *doṣas* and the three *guṇas*; this is made explicit by the commentator Ḍalhaṇa:

vyāsataḥ kīrtitaṃ tad dhi bhinnā doṣās trayo guṇaḥ
dviṣaṣṭidhā bhavanty ete bhūyiṣṭham iti niścayaḥ

For this has been proclaimed in detail: these faults, the
three *guṇas*, are mostly divided sixty-two-fold; that is the doctrine.

According to Ḍalhaṇa, wind consists mostly of *rajas*, because it promotes all beings, bile of *sattva*, because of its light and illuminating (fiery) nature, phlegm of *tamas*, because of its heavy and covering nature.[103]

As long as the three *guṇas* are in balance, they are not perceived;[104] the *guṇas* are mutually repressive.[105] Gauḍapāda on Sāṃkhya-kārikā 16 says: 'The Prime Materia is the state of equilibrium of *sattva*, *rajas*, and *tamas*' (*sattva-rajas-tamasāṃ sāmyâvasthā pradhānam*). The late compendium *Sarva-darśana-saṃgraha* (chapter 14) describes the evolution of the world as the move from *sāmyâvasthā* 'state of equilibrium' to *vaiṣamya* 'imbalance, inequality'.[106]

To sum up: Suśruta's intellectual achievement is the establishment of a homology of the three medical *doṣas* with the three ontological *guṇas* of Sāṃkhya; now the *doṣas* are permanent and necessary elements of a healthy body.

Aṣṭāṅga-saṃgraha and Aṣṭāṅga-hṛdaya-Saṃhitā

These two works ascribed to Vāgbhaṭa (often spelled Vāhaṭa)[107] may actually be the work of two authors, according to some scholars,[108] dubbed Vāgbhaṭa I and Vāgbhaṭa II. Of these the former would have flourished at about A.D. 600,[109] while the work of the latter(?) was quoted by an Arab author in A.D. 849/850 and must hence be earlier (perhaps 7th century).[110] Vāgbhaṭa is commonly counted as the third in the triad of great medical authorities — Caraka, Suśruta, Vāgbhaṭa.

AS Sū 1.40–42 gives the basic definitions of health and illness:

kālârtha-karmaṇāṃ yogo hīna-mithyâtimātrakaḥ
samyag-yogaś ca vijñeyo rogârogyaîka-kāraṇam
rogas tu doṣa-vaiṣamyaṃ doṣa-sāmyam arogatā
nijâgantu-vibhāgena rogāś ca dvi-vidhā matāḥ
teṣāṃ kāya-mano-bhedād adhiṣṭhānam api dvidhā
rajas tamaś ca manaso dvau ca doṣāv udāhṛtau

Diminished, wrong, or excessive application of time (season), objects or actions and the correct application [of these] is the only cause of illness and health. Illness is the imbalance of the faults, health the balance of the faults. And the illnesses are twofold by the division of being innate[111] or accidental.[112]

Of these [illnesses] the location is also twofold by the division of body and mind; and *rajas* and *tamas* are listed as the two faults of the mind.

These stanzas occur with only a minor variation[113] in *AHS* Sū 1.19–21, but the preceding line of the *AS* (39 *cd*) is omitted:

sattvaṃ rajas tamaś cêti trayaḥ proktā mahāguṇāḥ

sattva, *rajas*, and *tamas*: the three are called the great *guṇas*.

This line in the *AS* marks the transition from a discussion of various concepts of the *guṇa*s (such as heavy, soft, smooth, etc.,) to the causes of health and illness, putting the three *guṇa*s of Sāṃkhya in close proximity to the three *doṣa*s of medicine. But it is awkward that *rajas* and *tamas*, which have just been called 'great *guṇas*' in stanza 39, are called the *doṣa*s of the mind in stanza 42. The author of *AHS* avoided the awkwardness by simply omitting the reference to the 'great *guṇas*'.

S. Dasgupta[114] and P. Kutumbiah[115] noted correctly that Vāgbhama's definition of health as *doṣa-sāmya* and illness as *doṣa-vaiṣamya* replaces the definitions *dhātu-sāmya* and *dhātu-vaiṣamya*, but they overlooked the antecedents in the *Suśruta-saṃhitā*. Hence, Kutumbiah attributed this development to 'advancement in medical thought' rather than to the influence of philosophical speculation.

The three *guṇa*s of Sāṃkhya are compared to the three *doṣa*s of medicine in *AS* Sū 21.32:

> *ārambhakaṃ virodhe 'pi mitho yad yad guṇa-trayam*
> *viśvasya dṛṣṭaṃ yugapad vyādher doṣa-trayaṃ tathā*

> As the triad of *guṇa*s in spite of their mutual opposition
> is seen to set the universe in motion simultaneously, thus
> the triad of *doṣa*s [sets] disease [in motion]

and in *AS* Sū 22.5

> *doṣā eva hi sarva-rogaîka-kāraṇam. yathaîva śakuniḥ*
> *sarvataḥ paripatan divasaṃ svāṃ chāyāṃ nâtivartate,*
> *yathā vā kṛtsnaṃ vikāra-jātaṃ vaiśva-rūpyeṇa vyavasthi-*
> *taṃ guṇa-trayam apy atiricya na vartate, tathaîvêdam*
> *api kṛtsnaṃ vikāra-jātaṃ doṣa-trayam iti*

> The faults are the only cause of all illnesses. As a bird
> flying all over for a day does not go beyond its own
> shadow,[116] or as the transformed universe, established in
> all its forms does not exist beyond the three *guṇa*s, thus
> also all this that is transformed (i.e., illnesses) [does not
> exist beyond] the three *doṣa*s.[117]

Suśruta II and Ḍalhaṇa came close to identifying the three *doṣa*s with the three *guṇa*s; Vāgbhātā was satisfied with a homology that cemented the role of the *doṣa*s as basic constituents of the body.

'The body is based on the *doṣa*s, the elements, (and) the secretions', say both authors.[118] 'The *doṣa*s, if spoiled, spoil the elements through the tastes, both (spoil) the secretions'.[119] The elements can therefore be defined as *dūṣya* 'to be spoiled': 'The elements chyle, blood, flesh, fat, bone, marrow (and) semen are the seven *dūṣya*s, and also the secretions, i.e., urine, faeces, sweat, etc'.[120] The 'non-transformed', i.e., healthy *doṣa*s have their natural locations in the body: *iti prāyeṇa doṣāṇāṃ sthānāny avi-kṛtâtmanām* (*AHS* Sū 12.18). Caraka would have spoken of the natural location of wind, bile, and phlegm instead.[121]

To sum up: Vāgbhaṭa (and it does not matter whether he was two authors or one) presents the definite shape of the *tri-doṣa* theory. The three *doṣa*s are constant elements of the body; their equilibrium constitutes health, their imbalance illness.

Conclusion

We have traced the semantic development of *doṣa* in the (essentially) North Indian tradition where it first means an affliction — especially a pathological affliction of wind, bile, and phlegm — and then is a common term for these three components of the body. This happened under the influence of a perceived homology with the three *guṇa*s of the Sāṃkhya philosophy, at a time when the two Sanskrit words had become antonyms in general usage: *guṇa* 'quality, virtue', versus *doṣa* 'fault'. Beginning with Suśruta, and henceforth, three 'faults' are the basis of health. Indian medicine, rooted in popular observation and folk remedies, as we can still see in the earliest Buddhist canonical texts, had become a dogmatic system linked with a prestigious ideology. Caraka made a first (almost playful) attempt to link medicine with philosophy which had no major impact on his presentation of medicine; Suśruta perfected the homology and applied it rigorously to medical theory. Some formulations of Vāgbhaṭa became standard expressions in later texts. The commentators of the classical medical texts have worked hard, as was to be expected, to create a consistent system of Āyurvedic theory that neglects the changes that happened over time. For all their efforts they have trouble defining what exactly constitutes a *doṣa*.[122]

We find, on the other hand, no trace of an evolution in the Tamil tradition that would explain the odd concept of health being based on a balance of faults. We must conclude, then, that the medicine of the Tamil Cittars is based on the later development found in the works of Suśruta and Vāgbhaṭa, at least as far as their theory of the three faults is concerned. The discussion of cultural exchanges between Sanskritic and Tamil traditions must be removed from the highly charged atmosphere that has too often dominated such discussions over the past decades and should resort to the investigation of technical details. The present study is meant as a step in that direction, and it is my hope that my Tamil friends also will find its logic compelling. If it could elucidate at the same time the evolution of Āyurvedic theory, I would consider this a bonus.

Notes

1. This chapter is a reprint of the essay 'The Doctrine of the Three Humors in Traditional Indian Medicine and the Alleged Antiquity of Tamil Siddha Medicine', *Journal of the American Oriental Society*, vol. 119, no. 4, October–December 1999, pp. 609–629. Reproduced with permission. The style of reference citation has been retained as in the original article.
2. There can be little doubt that Tamil *cittar* is derived from Sanskrit *siddha*, with the Tamil suffix *-r* to denote plurality or respect. However, already the *Tēvāram* poets connected the word with Sanskrit *cit* or *citta* 'thought': R. Venkatraman, *A History of the Tamil Siddha Cult* (Madurai, 1990: 2f.), with reference to *Tēvāram* 6.46.3 and 5.76.5. This connection was very suggestive inasmuch the distinction of /tt/ and /ddh/ in the original Sanskrit was lost as these words were accepted as loans in Tamil.
3. There are government-supported institutions now in Madras and Palayamkotta and elsewhere for teaching, research, and treatment of patients, based on Siddha doctrine.
4. The *Tamil Lexicon* derives the (earlier) form Ciṟṟampalam from Skt. *cit*. This can hardly be correct; Ciṟṟampalam must contain the word for 'small' as in ciṟṟaṉiviṉār 'having little wisdom' (Nālaṭiyār 329.4). Ciṟṟamparam and Citambaram occur together in *Tirumantiram* 886 (866); for ref. see note 13. B. Natarajan, *Tirumantiram*, 141f., takes Ciṟṟampalam as a 'Tamilized form of Chidambaram'.
5. R. Manickavasagam gives further examples in 'Contribution of Agasthiyar to Siddha System of Medicine' *Heritage of the Tamils: Siddha Medicine*, ed. S. V. Subramanian and V. R. Madhavan (Madras, 1983: 582).
6. R. Venkatraman, *History*, 114, 179f. Cf. K. Zvelebil, *The Smile of Murugan* (Leiden, 1973: 223).
7. T. G. Ramamurthi Iyer, *The Hand Book of Indian Medicine: The Gems of Siddha System* (Erode, 1933; repr. Delhi, 1981), 13–15; A. Ramalingam and G. Veluchamy, 'Elements of Medical Science in Sangam Literature', in *Heritage of the Tamils: Siddha Medicine*, 44–53; K. and L. Palanichamy, *Heritage*, 550–67.
8. *Akanāṉūṟu*, ed. South India Saiva Siddhanta Works Publishing Society (1946 [1959]), nos. 133, 257; *Puṟanāṉūṟu*, ed. SISSWPS (Madras, 1947–51 [1959–62]), nos. 60, 170, 321.
9. Paripāṭal, ed. tr. F. Gros (Pondichéry, 1968), colophons of Paripāṭal 15 and 19.
10. Cilappatikāram, ed. SISSWPS (Madras, 1942; repr. [1966]).
11. *Lexicon of Tamil Literature* (Leiden, 1995: 146). The reference to king Gajabāhu of Ceylon is often taken as an indication that the work may have been composed around 200 A.D.; the historicity of Gajabāhu has been denied by G. Obeyesekere, most recently in his *The Cult of the Goddess*

Pattini (1984: 361–80), but defended by K. Zvelebil, *Tamil Literature* (1975: 38f.), and *Lexicon*, 145f. The final redaction of the text may, however, be somewhat later.

12. The Tirukkuṛaḷ of Tiruvalluvar is dated by K. Zvelebil about 450 to 550 A.D.: *Lexicon*, 669: cf. *The Sacred Kurral*, ed., tr. G. U. Pope (1886, repr. New Delhi [1984]).
13. Some interpreters have mistakenly assumed that it is food and work that increase or decrease: *Tirukkural*, tr. G. U. Pope, W. H. Drew, John Lazarus, and F. W. Ellis (Madras, 1958); A. Ramalingam and G. Veluchamy, *Heritage*, 50.
14. *Tirumantiram: A Tamil Scriptural Classic by Tirumular*, tr. B. Natarajan, 2nd ed. (Madras, 1994); *Tirumantiram*, ed. SISSWPS (1942; 8th ed., Madras, [1989]). The numbers of the latter edition are added in parentheses.
15. R. Manickavasagam, *Tirumantira ārāycci* (Madras, 1982), 74f.
16. R. Manickavasagam, *Tirumantira ārāycci*, 91; *Encyclopaedia of Tamil Literature*, I: 296 (J. Parthasarathi: sixth century); K. Zvelebil, *Tamil Literature*, 138; *Lexicon*, 677, suggests the late sixth or early seventh centuries.
17. I could not verify this reference in the editions of B. Natarajan or the SISSWPS, which contain only 3047 and 3001 stanzas, respectively.
18. Stanzas 740–69 (720–49).
19. *History*, 45–48.
20. R. Venkatraman assumes the existence of two men named Tirumūlar: one referred to in a ninth-century text, who may have been one of the sixty-three nāyanmār; the other, the author of the *Tirumantiram* in the tenth or eleventh century. A similar suggestion was already made by S. Vaiyapuri Pillai, *History of Tamil Language and Literature* (Madras, 1956: 108 n. 3).
21. S. Vaiyapuri Pillai, *History*, 108 n. 3; T. P. Meenakshisundaran, *A History of Tamil Literature* (Annamalainagar, 1965: 67); K. Zvelebil, *Tamil Literature*, 138.
22. R. Venkatraman, *History*, 45.
23. In the commentary on *Yāpparuṅkalam* 93, ed. M. V. Venugopala Pillai (Madras, 1960: 288): S. Vaiyapuri Pillai, *History*, 108; R. Venkatraman, *History*, 193.
24. There are references, though, to beliefs and practices found in a wider field, as R. Venkatraman, *History*, 145f. points out: The beliefs of the Siddhas in immortality, rejuvenation, finding God within the body through Yōga, the doctrine of *vāṉūṟal* (*sōmarasa* or "nectar in the body"), urine therapy, the eight great *siddhis*, sorcery and astrology are all traceable to the *Tirumandiram*.'
25. R. Venkatraman, *History*, 118f.
26. R. Venkatraman, *History*, 116.

27. R. Manickavasagam in Madras and S. Prema in Tanjore. This is also the opinion of T. P. Meenakshisundaran, according to K. Zvelebil, *The Poets of the Powers* (London, 1973: 71).
28. Thus the *Tamil Lexicon* under mukkuṟṟam, with reference to the Piṅkalanikaṇṭu. A group of six evils (*ari-ṣaḍ-varga*) is frequently encountered, e.g., *Arthaśāstra*, ed. R. P. Kangle (Bombay, 1960), 1.6.1: *kāma-krodha-lobha-māna-mada-harṣa*. K. and L. Palanichamy seem to assume that *mu-kkuṟṟam* refers here to the three humors *vaḷi*, *azhal*, and *īyam*: *Heritage*, 560 n. 1.
29. R. Venkatraman, *History*, 113, quotes the term as *nañcu* instead of *ai*, apparently by mistake.
30. R. Venkaraman, *History*, 118, quotes Tirumantiram 480 for the imbalance of humours; this stanza is probably the same as the one quoted here as 458, which may contain a vague allusion to the three *guṇa*s of Sāṃkhya but none of the terms denoting humours. The three *guṇa*s (*mu-kkuṇa*) are clearly mentioned in *Tirumantiram* 615 (595).
31. It is a pity that R. Venkatraman, *History*, 117, does not give references from the medical Siddha texts.
32. E.g., several contributors to the volume *Heritage of the Tamils*, 172, 185, 219; *Encyclopaedia of Tamil Literature*, I: 335.
33. Cf. *piṇi* 'disease' in Tirukkuṟaḷ stanzas 949 and 1102.
34. Cf. the critical remark made by R. Müller, *Sudhoffs Archiv für Geschichte der Medizin und der Naturwissenschaften* 32 (1939: 291).
35. In the title of the Hippocratic text *περί χμῶν* 'Humours': *The Loeb Classical Library: Hippocrates*, vol. IV, tr. W. H. S. Jones (Cambridge, Mass., 1931[1998]: 62).
36. E.g., in the hippocratic text *Nature of Man*, ch. 4f.; *Hippocrates*, 10–13.
37. *Asceticism and Healing in Ancient India* (New York, 1991).
38. There seems to be some corruption in the second line of this śloka: both quarters have nine syllables, and the feminine form *atthamī* is out of place; shall one emend to *visamam, opakkamikam, kamma-vipāko aṭṭhamo 'ti*?
39. P. Demiéville, '"*Byō*" *from Hōbōgirin*', tr. M. Tatz (Lanham, Md., 1985: 71). Several passages discussed by Demiéville on pp. 65–76 point to a struggle to reconcile a Buddhist doctrine of four constituent elements of the body (earth, water, fire, wind) with the concept of the three causes of illness, i.e., bile, phlegm, and wind.
40. Also *Cullavagga* V.14.1 = *Vin* II.119.
41. R. Müller, *Janus* 38 (1934: 80).
42. K. G. Zysk, *Asceticism*, 108f., 124f.
43. The 'sickness of the hot season' (*sāradika-ābādha MV* VI. 1 = *Vin* 1.199, where only the much later commentator Buddha-ghosa suggests bile as the cause), the 'disease of thick scabs' (*thulla-kacchâbādha MV* VI.9 = *Vin* 1.202), 'disease of the eyes' (*cakkhu-rogâbāha MV* VI. 11 = *Vin* 1.203), 'heat

in the head' (*sīsâbhitāpa MV* VI. 13 = *Vin* 1.204), boils (*gaṇḍâbādhaMV* VI. 14 + *Vin* 1.205), constipation (*dummha-gahaṇika MV* VI.14 = *Vin* 1.206), jaundice (*pāṇḍu-rogâbādha*, ibid.), skin disease (*chavi-dosâbādha*, ibid.), fistula-in-ano (*bhagandlâbādha MV* VI.22 = *Vin* 1.215).

44. *Asceticism*, 76; cf., also p. 110.
45. See n. 40.
46. Cf., G. J. Meulenbeld, 'The Characteristics of a *Doṣa*', *Journal of the European Ayurvedic Society* 2 (1992): 1.
47. Cf., K. Zysk, 'The Evolution of Anatomical Knowledge in Ancient India, with Special Reference to Cross-Cultural Influences', *JAOS* 106 (1986: 689).
48. This list is found also in *Majjhima-nikāya* 1.57 and III.90f. (with further elaboration on the following pages) and, without reference to the *dhātus*, in *Aṅguttara-nikāya* III.323f. A bare list is found in *Khuddakapāṭha* 3 (*Khuddaka-nikāya*, PTS ed., I.2); cf., also *Sutta-nipāṭha*. 195–201 (*Khuddaka-nikāya*, PTS ed., p. 34f.).
49. The relative frequency of wind as a cause of illness in the texts quoted by Zysk does not support F. Zimmermann's theory that wind was 'grafted onto the humoral theory at a later stage' while 'its core concepts, *bile* and *phlegm*, stem from cosmology', Review of K. Zysk, *Asceticism*, *JAOS* 113 (1993: 322). But bile and phlegm at the root of Hippocratic nosology (i.e., in the presumably older texts) offer, indeed, a remarkable parallel.
50. Ed. F. Kielhorn, 3rd ed. (Poona, 1965), II: 351.7–14.
51. J. Filliozat, *The Classical Doctrine of Indian Medicine*, tr. Dev Raj Chanana (Delhi, 1964: 192), goes too far when he asserts that Kātyāyana's *vārttika* 'fully assures us that the pathological theory of the *tridoṣa* . . . had been fully constituted in Kātyāyana's time'.
52. R. P. Das, 'Miscellanea de Operibus Āyurvedicis (II)', *Journal of the European Āyurvedic Society* 2 (1992: 27–29).
53. *The Bower Manuscript*, ed., tr. A. F. R. Hoernle (Calcutta, 1893–1912). Quotations refer to the stanzas of the texts.
54. Lore Sander, in *Investigating Indian Art*, ed. M. Yaldiz and W. Lobo (Berlin, 1987: 313–23); and similar already, A. H. Dani, *Indian Palaeography* (Oxford, 1963: 151).
55. R. Müller, *Grundsätze altindischer Medizin* (Copenhagen, 1951: 120), rightly criticises Hoernle's translation of *doṣa* as 'humour' rather than 'Fehler' in the texts of the Bower Manuscript.
56. J. Jolly, *ZDMG* 53 (1899: 379); idem, *Indian Medicine*, tr. C. G. Kashikar (Poona, 1951: 60f).
57. At least some of the Vedic evidence deals with the body of the sacrificial animal.
58. This ambiguity may reflect a phase in the development of Āyurveda when the role of the three faults in nosology was not yet fixed, as G. J. Meulenbeld has suggested: 'The Constraints of Theory in the Evolution

of Nosological Classifications: A Study on the Position of Blood in Indian Medicine (Āyurveda)', in *Medical Literature from India, Sri Lanka, and Tibet*, ed. G. J. Meulenbeld, Panels of the VIIth World Sanskrit Conference (Leiden, 1991), 8–9: 91–106.

59. Cf., earlier sections in this chapter.
60. H. Lüders, *Philologica Indica* (Göttingen, 1940: 586–88); a new edition and translation is found in R. Müller, *Grundsätze altindischer Medizin*, 40f.
61. *Buddhacaritam*, ed. E. H. Johnston (Lahore, 1936; repr. Delhi [1984]). Aśvaghoṣa, the author of the *Buddhacarita*, is usually assumed to have lived in the first or second century A.D.
62. *The Sūtra of Golden Light, Being a Translation of the Suvarṇabhāsottama-sūtra* (by) R. E. Emmerick (London, 1970), 75f. The Sanskrit text was not available to me. Emmerick (p. ix) dates the text approximately at the beginning of the fifth century A.D. (when it was translated into Chinese). The compilation of the text stretched over several centuries, and there are numerous versions. J. Nobel proposes A.D. 300 as the approximate date of the nucleus of this medical chapter: *Ein alter medizinischer Sanskrit-Text und seine Deutung*, supplement to *JAOS* 71 (1951: 34).
63. J. Nobel, *Ein alter medizinischer Sanskrit-Text*, 11.
64. In its present form the text contains some expressions that can hardly be earlier than the early centuries A.D. In Sū 12.8 we find the poetic expression *an-oka-ha* 'tree' (lit. 'not leaving its home'), which is otherwise attested only in Kālidāsa's *Raghuvaṃśa* 2.13 and a version of the *Śakuntalā* (so *PW*); *an-oka-sārī* 'not living in his home, beggar' is found in *Mahābhārata* I 86.5; *mṛdvīkā* 'grape' (Sū 25.49) is a wrong sanskritisation of a loan word from Iranian *madvīka* (literature in H. Scharfe, *Investigations in Kautalya's Manual of Political Science* [Wiesbaden 1993: 88]). Such late words may point to insertions or reformulations of the text.
65. *Car* Ci 30.289f. and Si 12.36–40.
66. A. F. R. Hoernle, *JRAS* 1908: 997–1028; G. J. Meulenbeld, *The Mādhavanidāna* (Leiden, 1974: 411); Debiprasad Chattopadhyaya, *Science and Society in Ancient India* (Calcutta, 1977: 31–33); H. Scharfe, 'The Language of the Physician', in *Fs. G. Cardona* (forthcoming).
67. Cf., *Mahābhārata* XII.330.21f. In *Car* Vi 8.95 again 'excessive *doṣas*' cause the above mentioned unhealthy dispositions; those with balanced *dhātus* are endowed with all good qualities (Vi 8.100). Even centuries later, *Aṣṭāṅga-hṛdaya* Sū 1.10 retains the distinction of the ideal *sama-dhātuḥ* [*prakṛtiḥ*] and the undesirable disposition caused by faults (*doṣa*); it is only Aruṇadatta, in his commentary on this stanza, who maintains that *doṣa* here (!) is nothing but a synonym of *dhātu*: *dhātu-śabdo 'tra doṣa-paryāyaḥ*.
68. H. Scharfe, *The State in Indian Tradition* (Leiden, 1989: 2: 28 n. 18).
69. The commentator, Cakrapāṇi, explains that this problem can be avoided if measures are taken during the rainy season that prevents the build-up of bile.

70. *Vātâdayaḥ prakupyanti śirasy asraṃ ca duṣyati*
tataḥ śirasi jāyante rogā vividha-lakṣaṇāḥ | 11 |
71. 'Being riled, riles' is expressed in various similar ways: *kupyati*, *prakupyanti*, *atikopayati* (Sū 26.84), etc.
72. *Śiro-gatāḥ sirā vṛddho vāyur āviśya kupyati*
tataḥ śūlaṃ mahat tasya vātāt samupajāyate | 18 |
73. *Kamv-amla-lavaṇa-kṣāra-madya-krodhâtapānalaiḥ*
pittaṃ śirasi saṃduṣṭaṃ śiro-rogāya kalpate | 22 |
74. *Āsyā-sukhaiḥ svapna-sukhair guru-snigdhātibhojanaiḥ*
śleṣmā śirasi saṃduṣṭaḥ śiro-rogāya kalpate | 24 |
75. In Sūtra-sthāna 1.59–61 we find side by side *saṃpraśāmyati*, *praśāmyati*, and *praśamaṃ yānti*. By metonymy an illness can also be 'calmed': 'by an oil-massage the body becomes one in whom the wind-disease is calmed', i.e., not susceptible to diseases due to wind (Sū 5.86 *śarīram abhyaṅgād . . . jāyate praśānta-mārutâbādhaṃ*).
76. A certain 'oil is killing the three faults' (*tailam etad tridoṣa-ghnam*): Sū 5.70.
77. Sū 10.11, 13.
78. *Tri-doṣa-ja* is also found in Sū 17.26, but here it may refer to a headache caused by any of the three *doṣa*s individually.
79. *Saṃnipāta* also occurs several times in Sū 19.4.
80. In Sū 5.6 *doṣa* is not used in its technical sense: 'light [articles of food] are of little harm (*alpa-doṣāṇi*) even if taken in excess . . . heavy [articles of food] are exceedingly harmful (*doṣavanti*)'.
81. *Caraka Saṃhitā*, tr. Ram Karan Sharma and Vaidya Bhagwan Dash (Benares, 1976), I: 106.
82. S. Chidambarathanu Pillai, *Siddha System of Diseases* (Madras, 1992), ii f.
83. J. Filliozat (*The Classical Doctrine*, 28 and 187) also speaks of the three elements (*tridhātu*) which become the three troubles (*tridoṣa*) when they are disturbed; but he does not elaborate on the use of these terms in earlier and later Āyurvedic texts.
84. According to Cakrapāṇi, the reference is to faeces, etc., and chyle, etc.
85. These almost untranslatable terms denote two of the three strands (*guṇa*) that make up the prime materia in classical Sāṃkhya doctrine; *rajas* 'sky, dusk, redness, defilement, passion' denotes a restless, active element; *tamas* 'darkness' a dull, sluggish element. The third is *sattva* 'createdness, living being; goodness', an element of brightness, knowledge, and capacity of release: J. A. B. van Buitenen, *JAOS* 77 (1957: 88–107). One can define the three *guṇa*s functionally: 'The subtle matter of pure thought or *sattva*, the kinetic matter of pure energy or *rajas*, and the reified matter of inertia or *tamas*', see G. J. Larson, *Philosophy East and West* 37 (1987): 249. Cf., R. Müller, *Janus* 38 (1934): 77–93.
86. The desire to find homologies is also noticeable in *Car* Sū 12.13 where *vāta*, *pitta*, and *śleśman* in their proper and their disturbed states are compared

to the proper and improper attendance to the three goals in life (*dharma, artha, kāma*) and to the three seasons, whose 'unseasonal' weather spells disaster.

87. This passage invalidates the statement by P. Kutumbiah, *Ancient Indian Medicine* (Bombay, 1962: 73), that 'Caraka does not mention the guṇas at all in connection with the *doṣas*'. On some linkage of the medical *doṣas* and the philosophical *guṇas* of Sāṃkhya, cf., Arion Roşu, *Les Conceptions psychologiques dans les textes médicaux indiens* (Paris, 1978: 108, 118, 192).
88. Cf. S. N. Dasgupta, *A History of Indian Philosophy* (Cambridge, 1922; repr. Delhi [1975]), I: 216; E. H. Johnston, *Early Sāṃkhya* (London, 1937 repr. Delhi [1974]: 35); E. Frauwallner, *WZKM* 32 (1925: 188 ff.); J. A. B. van Buitenen, *JAOS* 77 (1957: 99 ff.); G. Larson, *Classical Sāṃkhya*, 2nd ed. (Delhi, 1979: 45, 112, 131, 162–64).
89. Cf. S. Dasgupta, *A History of Indian Philosophy*, I: 126.
90. *Sattva* is used in widely divergent contexts and meanings: van Buitenen, *JAOS* 77 (1957: 95–99).
91. Some Indian traditions recognised four origins of life, lit. 'wombs', viz., chorion, egg, sweat (insects, etc.), sprouts (plants).
92. The absence of a common term for healthy wind, bile, and phlegm in the older texts necessitates frequent enumeration of all three (as in Sū 7.39) or abbreviation (*vātâdayaḥ* Sū 17.11, *pittâdīnām* Sū 17.114).
93. This vital force is considered to reside in the heart: J. Filliozat, *The Classical Doctrine*, 27f., 166f. with reference to Caraka, Sū 30.6–11.
94. Cf. Bhela-saṃhitā, ed. V. S. Venkatasubramania Sastri and C. Raja Rajeswara Sarma (1977), Sū 26.34:

    yathā patatriḥ śīghro 'pi svāṃ chāyāṃ nâtivartate
    vātâder [read vātâdīn] nātivartante bahavo 'pi tathâmayāḥ

    As a bird — even a fast one — does not transgress its shadow, thus even the diseases — even in their multitude — do not transgress wind, etc.

    In a different category are afflictions caused by external forces, such as a blow: *Car* Sū 19.6.
95. The *Bhela-saṃhitā*, which had been eclipsed for a long time, has been recovered, though in imperfect textual condition (see n. 93). It is assumed to be of comparable antiquity with the works of Caraka and Suśruta. A cursory study showed that ill-applied heat riles wind, which in turn agitates the *doṣas* — all three *doṣas* then spoil the blood (Ci 6.8f.); dysentery caused by mental anguish leads to a riled *doṣa* (Ci 10.42); undigested food leads to riled elements (*dhātu*), and the force of these *doṣas* is increased by wind (Ci 10.51). Here Bhela seems to agree with Caraka in that *vāta*,

pitta, and *sleṣman* are only called *doṣa*s in their abnormal state. Only in a corrupt passage (Ci 20.3) do we find *doṣâsātmya* [sic] 'imbalance of faults'.

96. J. Filliozat, *The Classical Doctrine*, 273, also considers the section on prognostics in *Suśruta*, Sūtra-sthāna, chapters 29 to 33, as an improvement on Caraka's and Bhela's Indriya-sthāna.

97. H. Zimmer, *Hindu Medicine* (Baltimore, 1979; repr. New York [1948]: 134), is typical for the lax manner in which translators insert the term 'humor' with no textual basis in works on Āyurveda: 'The three humors, wind, bile, and phlegm are the basis of the existence of the human body'.

98. Cf. *Aṣṭāṅga-saṃgraha* Sū 20.1. The closest parallel is found in Mahābhārata V.33.81, where the body is called *tri-sthūṇa*; in the Bower manuscript, *Nāvanītaka* 500, 'fever is based on the three pillars' (*tri-sthūṇa-gatam . . .jvaram*). I do not, so far, understand the image of a house resting on three poles.

99. Blood is a cause of disease only as an intermediary; for it is itself 'aggravated by wind . . . aggravated by bile . . . and aggravated by phlegm . . . aggravated by a combination [of all three] or joined [by two of them] (Sū 14.21 *vātena duṣṭam . . . pitta-duṣṭam . . . śleṣma-duṣṭañ ca . . . sannipāta-duṣṭam . . . saṃ-sṛṣṭam*). Cakrapāṇi on *Caraka* Sū 1.57 notes that the seeming inclusion of blood among the *doṣa*s in *Car* Sū 24.18 and Ci 5.27 does not make it a fourth *doṣa*, as it itself is aggravated by wind, bile, or phlegm.

100. Deficiency in faeces, urine, and sweat is, if not perhaps a cause, at least a symptom; measures are taken to produce more stool and urine and to stimulate perspiration in Sū 15.11; cf., also *Caraka* Sū 17.70f.

101. G. J. Larson, *Philosophy East and West* 37 (1987: 258), seems to have overlooked this passage when he ascribed the postulation of this correspondence to Ḍalhaṇa (comm. on Uttara-tantra 66.9, numbered 66.6 in some editions, as in that quoted by Larson). There is a problem, as Larson points out, that *vāta*, *pitta*, and *kapha* should all be derived from *tamas* since they emerge from the *mahābhūtas*. The increasing emphasis on philosophical speculation in the medical schools and simultaneous de-emphasis or outright ban on experimentation led to stagnation in Indian medicine: Debiprasad Chattopadhyaya, *Science and Society in Ancient India* (1977: 157f). The veterinary work *Hasty-āyurveda* localises *sattva* in the phlegm, *rajas* in the wind, and *tamas* in the bile: Arion Roşu, *Les Conceptions psychologiques*, 118.

102. J. Filliozat, *The Classical Doctrine*, 12; G. J. Meulenbeld, *The Mādhavanidāna* (1974: 431f).

103. *Rajo-bhūyiṣṭho mārutaḥ, rajo hi pravartakaṃ sarva-bhāvānaṃ, pittaṃ sattvôtkaṭaṃ laghu-prakāśakatvāt, rajo-yuktaṃ vā ity eke kaphas tamo-bahulaḥ, guru-prāvaraṇâtmakatvād ity āhur bhiṣajaḥ.* The text is quoted from S. Dasgupta, *A History of Indian Philosophy* (1932), II: 329 n. 3.

104. E. Frauwallner, *Geschichte der indischen Philosophie*, 1: 308, 353.

105. *Sāṃkhya-kārikā* 12: *anyonyâbhibhavâśraya-janana-mithuna-vṛttayaś ca guṇāḥ* 'The strands mutually domineer, rest on each other, produce each other, consort together, and are reciprocally present'.
106. *Sāṃkhya-kārikā* 46 traces the varieties of ignorance, etc., to the 'destructive influence of the imbalance of the strands (*guṇa-vaiṣamya-vimarda*)'.
107. C. Vogel (*Vāgbhaṭa's Aṣṭāṅgahṛdayasaṃhitā* 1965: 45) discusses the various attested forms of the name.
108. C. Vogel (*Vigbhaṭa's Aṣṭāṅgahṛdayasaṃhitā*, 1–10) and G. J. Meulenbeld (*The Mādhavanidāna*, 423–25) review the arguments for and against the assumption of one or two Vāgbhaṭas, leaning towards a belief in only one author; the problem has little relevance for the present investigation, since both texts differ little concerning the topics under discussion. The *AS* is apparently the later work (or a later recension of the *AHS*), but not necessarily by another author.
109. G. J. Meulenbeld, *The Mādhavanidāna*, 423–25.
110. F. Filliozat, *The Classical Doctrine*, 14; G. J. Meulenbeld, *The Mādhavanidāna*, 425.
111. I.e., caused by *doṣas* linked to faulty nutrition or behaviour.
112. I.e., caused by external forces, such as a fall, an injury which brings about an imbalance of wind, bile, and phlegm (*Car* Sū 20.7) resulting in illness.
113. The last *pāda* of *AHS* Sū 1.20 differs in form, though not in content, from *AS* Sū 1.41: *tatra rogā dvidhā smṛtāḥ.*
114. S. Dasgupta, *A History*, II: 328.
115. P. Kutumbiah, *Ancient Indian Medicine*, 60f.
116. Cf. *Caraka* Sū 19.5 and *Bhela* Sū 26.34 (above pp. 624–25), where however, there is no reference to the *guṇas* of Sāṃkhya! In *AS* and *AHS kṛtsnaṃ vikārajātam* seems to be the agent, *guṇa-trayam* and *doṣa-trayam* the object, which is similar to the construction in *Car* Sū 19.5 (*sarve vikārā vāta-pitta-kaphān nâti-vartante*); *Su* Sū 24.8 has it the other way around: *kṛtsnaṃ vikāra-jātam . . . avyatiricya vāta-pitta-śleṣmāṇo vartante.*
117. *Aṣṭāṅga-hṛdaya* Sū 12.32–34 says essentially the same, except that it inserts the imbalance of the three elements (*dhātu*) as an intermediate cause:

tathā sva-dhātu-vaiṣamya-nimittam api sarvadā
vikāra-jātam trīn doṣān (supply: *nâtivartate*) |34|

118. *AS* Sū 19.1 *doṣa-dhātu-mala-mūlo hi dehaḥ* and *AHS* Sū 11.1 *doṣa-dhātu-malā mūlaṃ sadā dehasya.*
119. *AS* Sū 19.14 *cd* = *AHS* Sū 11.35 *cd*
doṣā duṣṭā rasair dhātūn dūṣayanty ubhaye malān
120. *AS* Sū 1.29 = *AHS* Sū 1.13
rasâsṛṅ-māṃsa-medo-'sthi-majja-śukrāṇni dhātavaḥ
sapta dūṣyā malā mūtra-śakṛt-svedâdayo 'pi ca

121. It is remarkable that *AS* Sū 20.5 in this instance is closer to Caraka: *evam amīṣu sthāneṣu bhūyiṣṭham avikṛtāḥ sakala-śarīra-vyāpino 'pi vāta-pitta-sleṣmāṇo vartante.* We have to assume that these vast compilations incorporated elements from different periods and did not always achieve consistency.

122. G. J. Meulenbeld, *Journal of the European Ayurvedic Society* 2 (1992: 1–5).

Eight

The Body in the System of Medicine

Caraka and Harvey

Anuradha Veeravalli

The significance of the chapter on *sarirasthanam* (the foundation of the body) in the *Carakasamhita* becomes evident only when comparing and contrasting it with the principles of the new post-Enlightenment system of medicine, which came to be established with the publication and success of William Harvey's *De Motu Cordis* (*The Circulation of the Blood*) in 1628. The latter established with decisiveness the effectiveness of the principles of scientific method, experiment and analysis, of a new science for modern times.

Working within the anatomical tradition of medicinal science of the European Enlightenment, Harvey's method rested on his adoption of (*a*) vivisection as a method of scientific investigation; (*b*) 'autopsia' or 'seeing for oneself' as a principle of observation, that established the truth of the matter without doubt once and for all; and (*c*) objectivity determined by the possibility of public demonstration. Harvey held public demonstrations of dissection to prove his theories right. He consciously denied any association with philosophy, as did his contemporaries, who argued that anatomy, and not philosophy, was the basis of medicine. He saw his scientific method as being theory-neutral, based on evidence, and seen with his own eyes. However, his method of anatomical investigation presupposed, as does modern medicine, the clear separation of psychology, physiology and anatomy as three distinct areas of investigation in medicine, whose independent results could be used to assist one another in their understanding of the body and its workings. Harvey's anatomical work was followed by that of Pierre Cabanis on the influence of the psychological on the physical, and by Claude Bernard the physiologist in the 19th century, who discussed the relation of the internal environment of the body (homeostasis) to health. There appears, therefore, a clear division of labour, anticipating and following the Cartesian dualistic method, separating the trinity of mind and body, and mind and the external world.

This, then, constitutes the epistemological and metaphysical presupposition implicit in the method and classification that Harvey adopts: mind, body, and the external form of the body can, and are, studied separately. In fact, the anatomical method of Harvey set the ground for the classification and study of the body, organ by organ — a classification that seems to come naturally, self-evidently, to not only the practice of medicine, but also to our own understanding of the body today. Harvey begins his discussion on the circulation of blood by clearly demarcating the functions of the lung (vital element) and the heart (psychic element), which were earlier attributed together to constitute pulse. Pulsation, as he would demonstrate by vivisection, was merely due to the muscular movement of the heart. A quick check on the status of the relation between the lungs and the heart as it stands today reveals, however, that in times of a heart or a lung collapse, the most reliable first aid is still the CPR or cardio-pulmonary resuscitation. So, in spite of all autopsy results, it is the combination of the two that is critical for revival healing. Second, he held that there was no point to be made by saying that blood was spirituous; it was blood, whichever way. That he ignored what was at issue here will become clear in our discussion of La Mettrie.

Julien Ofray de La Mettrie (1709–51) was perhaps the lone figure amongst physicians in the 18th century to hold the view that physiologists are not only philosophers, but that they are also the only ones fit to be so. He got into trouble for these views and in 1748, lost his job and was given refuge by Fredrick the Great. The spiritualists disliked what they saw as heretic epicurean tendencies in his position, which stated that the body and the external world are signs of the spirit. The doctors thought of him as a philosopher whose abilities in medicine were doubtful, if not outdated. Fredrick thought he was a good man, a fine physician, but a bad writer. Clearly, the man of religion and the man of science seemed not only to uphold the separation of the world and the spirit, but to also defend it against all those who believed otherwise. Cartesian dualism had been established as the science and religion of the Enlightenment, and the body as the temple of God was as much a heresy in modern science as it was in modern religion.

La Mettrie did continue to fight in defence of the body as a sign of the non-dualism of mind/spirit and the world. He presented his theory in two lucid tracts — *Man: A Machine* and *Man: A Plant*. In the former, in a tongue-in-cheek retort of sorts to Descartes, he argued that the body of man was indeed a machine as Descartes would have it; only, it was a perpetual one, since the body working in conjunction with the soul was autonomous, and therefore perpetual.

He insisted that his theory of medicine and the body also depended on observation, experience and experiment. The difference was that his observations brought him to the conclusion that there could be no study of the functions of the animated body without the study of the soul. Consequently, it was only physicians who were philosophers, and who could truly be theologians. His method did not require the dissection of the body or an organ, but a keen observation of key signs of the relation of body and soul: sleep, food — essential for the nourishment and rejuvenation of the soul — the facility for reproduction, countenance, and speech — the unique condition that we know only through the constitution of signs by the act of co-relation of word and the world, that animals and men exhibited in varying degrees.

Here, one might briefly refer to his method of analysis. For instance, with respect to sleep, he argues in *Man: A Machine*:

> The soul and the body fall asleep together. As the motion of the blood is calmed, a sweet feeling of peace and quiet spreads through the whole mechanism. The soul feels itself little by little growing heavy as the eyelids droop, and loses its tenseness, as the fibres of the brain relax; thus little by little it becomes as if paralyzed and with it all the muscles of the body. These can no longer sustain the weight of the head, and the soul can no longer bear the burden of thought; it is in sleep as if we were not (1912: 31).

Two points need to be emphasised: (*a*) the relation between body and soul is clearly demonstrated as not being one of cause and effect — the soul is calm, therefore one sleeps. The relation is mutual, complementary — a matter of balance; (*b*) blood is what mediates between soul and body; it is the sign of their relationship. Thus, as the motion of blood calms, the whole mechanism is calmed. (This perhaps helps to explain Harvey's predecessors' insistence on 'spirituous blood'.)

The *Sarirasthanam* section in the *Carakasamhita* presents a particularly interesting study of the relation between science and religion,[1] since it disallows the separation of the two disciplines, once again much to the discomfort of both the spiritualist and the scientist. The body as object of study in the theory of longevity is the seat of the union of self/spirit and matter. Caraka argues that the sense organs that make possible the experience of pain and pleasure, life and death prove this fact, since there can be no pain with mere matter. Nor is the self known in this world without embodiment, which enables the experience of pain and pleasure. Thus, the section on the body is in effect a section on the 'impersonation' of the self. I use 'impersonation' instead of 'embodiment', since here, unlike in the Advaitic tradition, there is no one universal Self that appears as differentiated in this world. Rather, it is the selves that initiate a variety of conceptions, dispositions, and actions in undifferentiated *prakriti*. The person is then the sign, or rather, the symptom, of health, or the lack of it. Alternately, one may say that s/he is a cause/origin of these symptoms, so that at the point of conception, where semen and ovum meet, the self intervenes:

> There, first of all the principle of consciousness comes forward along with psyche to receive the qualities (of *mahabhutas*/elements — ether, air, fire, earth and water). He is *hetu, karana, nimitta* (sign, or cause of the sign),* *akshara* (undecaying), *karta* (doer), *manta* (thinker), *vedita* (preceptor), *boddha* (knower), *drshta* (seer), *dharta* (sustainer), *brahma* (creator), *vishwakarma* (craftsman of the Universe),* *vishwarupa* (form of the universe),* *purusa* (in the body), *prabhava* (source), *avyaya* (undamageable), *nitya* (eternal), *guni* (with qualities), *grahana* (to wear, assume, seize),* *pradhana* (principal), *avyakta* (unmanifest), *jiva* (life-principle), *jna* (conscious), *pudgala* (ego), *chetanavan* (having consciousness), *vibhu* (all pervasive),* *bhutatma* (essence of creatures), *indriyatma* (essence of sense organs), *and antaratma* (inner essence) . . . . At the time of putting on the (qualities and) body also, he takes up *aakasa* [ether] itself first of all and then the other four elements, with other manifest qualities gradually (*Sarirasthanam* IV: 8).[2]

The *Sarirasthanam* uses the terms *linga*, *karana*, *hetu*, *chinha* and *rupa* to express this notion of symptom in the text. Only a closer reading would clarify the technical difference, if any, in their usage. However, as in La Mettrie, the factors that combine to create the embryo — parents, nutrition, suitability, and self — are not 'causally' linked to the embryo. Caraka makes a considerable effort to clarify this point. It is rather their *samyoga* that the embryo is a sign of.

The self in the womb acquires her/his body and sense organs simultaneously. Thus, it attains 'a free flow of consciousness'. At this point, the embryo comes into being, pulsates, and has desires of its own. In effect, a person is born, and Caraka describes this state of the embryo as the state of two hearts — one, its own and the other, its mother's, through which it transmits its desires. Perhaps this is why, traditionally, the date of birth is counted from the day of conception, rather than the day of separation from the umbilical cord.

This focus on the body as 'impersonating' the self is fundamentally different from the orthodox understanding of the relation between body and self in Indian philosophy — the need for the self's emancipation from the body. It may be argued, however, that Caraka's understanding has its basis in the cosmological traditions of *Samkhya* and *Yoga*, and perhaps Ramanuja, who anticipates the metaphysical foundations of the Bhakti traditions that arise after the 12th century. In the study of both macrocosmic and microcosmic cosmologies, what is often lost sight of while focusing our attention on the principles of *purusa* and *Prakriti*, or mind and the external world, is the *linga*, sign of the union of *purusa* and *Prakriti*, and object of meditation in *Yoga*. This fact, though, is not missed in vernacular representations, where the *linga* is central to the truth of 'impersonation' and is by no means a sign of an illusory union, or illusory manifestation, as the Sanskritist or Brahminic orthodoxy would have it. In Caraka, the *linga* is a symptom — sign and measure — of the well-being, and therefore the healthy union, of self and body and self and the external world, known through the sense organs, the mind, and the will: 'The mind is characterised by knowledge arising from the presence or absence of contact between self and the sense organs. In connection with the mind, knowledge makes its presence' (*Sarirasthanam* I: 18–19).

The text goes on to explain that this knowledge is supplied to the *buddhi* (will), where its validity is decided and then acted upon.

The *Sarirasthanam* locates the union of mind and matter/the external world in the body, so that in effect, the real object of study in its system of medicine is the person/*purusa*. The body and its modifications — due to internal and external factors — form the symptoms that reveal the nature and state of this relation of the self and *mahabhutas*. This theory of symptomatology clearly depends on principles of investigation and a semiotic theory that is fundamentally different from those of modern science and philosophy. The body is not divided up into parts and organs, but into signs and symptoms that govern the relation between the self and different parts of the body, the self and its rejuvenation in the body, the self and its reproduction. The first chapter, on *indriyasthanam* (symptomatology), significantly discusses complexion and voice (and perhaps, in literate cultures, one could add handwriting!). The chapters that follow discuss the critical signs of life and death, health and disease in the sense organs pertaining to taste, touch, sight, mind, body (and its shadow/inverted image), bile, sputum, stool and semen.

Since the foetus, apart from its other qualities, is constituted of the five elements, Caraka holds that a person is equal to the universe, and vice versa. Whatever forms exist in the universe are also found in the person. ('Sarirasthanam', V: 3): 'When *yoga* is accomplished, *samkhya* is attained' (*Sarirasthanam* V: 16–19).

Gandhiji's own experiments with medicine, or what he called 'nature cure', involved a conscious distancing from the intricacies of Ayurveda. He was clear that what he called 'nature cure' was meant neither to sell a cure, nor to promise one. It was merely meant to initiate one into a life suited to nature — his own and that of the universe around him — and was not a form of treatment. With an almost uncanny knack for gauging the pulse of every aspect of the alternate modernity he wanted to present, Gandhi seemed to have picked the quintessence of Caraka's medicine. In his *Key to Health*, one of the four manuscripts he undertook to write as a book, he picks the five elements, the sun, food/diet, and *brahmacharya* as the four principles that determine healing and health. Like Caraka, he says, 'The human body is the Universe in miniature' (1992: 13).

The next difference with Ayurveda lies in Gandhiji's emphasis on the body as an instrument of service for the rest of creation, rather than an emphasis on emancipation per se. When the unity of the person and the universe is realised through service, the body becomes a temple worthy to live in. We are guardians/trustees of our body so that it may serve the body politic and the cosmos. This understanding of the body and focus on service directly addresses and mediates the post-Enlightenment Cartesian dualisms of mind and the world, mind and body, or matter and spirit. The body in the labour of production and reproduction, with the use of reason, skill and the will, in the act of service to another is witness to the relation between these dualisms. This, therefore, is the basis of Gandhiji's critique of modern Western civilisation, its back- and soul-breaking division of labour between workers of the mind and of the body. That he meant this to be so is proved not only by his advocating *khadi*, but also by the fact that he persuaded his nephew to start a technical journal in Hindi to discuss the problems of the *charkha*, innovation, and so on — a veritable R&D institution in the vernacular.

However, his best contribution to the cause of science and religion is his appropriation of the term *ashram* — a term that refers traditionally to an institution considered a place of retreat — to the cause of his experiments with truth. He reinstituted the term 'ashram' in its rightful place in a new modernity, recapturing at once its etymological lineage in the term *shram*, meaning 'labour', albeit with self-reflection, thus placing it at the fore and beside the term 'laboratory', whose root also derives from 'labour'. There was a fundamental difference, however, since the *ashram* was meant to conduct experiments with truth, that is, with signs and sites of the union of mind/spirit and the world, while the laboratory conducted experiments concerning the dualism of the two, discovering and establishing their separate and different truths.

Acknowledgement

Discussions with Punam Zutshi have helped immensely in formulating the structure of arguments in this chapter.

Notes

1. I prefer the opposition of science and religion to the opposition of science and spirituality, since the former does not necessarily presume the separation of matters of science and matters of the spirit. As I have tried to argue, both science and religion prior to the European Enlightenment constitute the nature of the body and the cosmos as signs of the union of matter and spirit, instead of reducing them to objects in the external world that stand in opposition to the spirit or consciousness.
2. I have translated the asterisked terms differently from P. V. Sharma, whose translation of *Carakasamhita* has been cited here, since it seemed more appropriate to the overall meaning of the text that talks of the 'impersonation' of the self.

References

de La Mettrie, Julien Offray. 1912. *Man a Machine* (Gertrude Carman Bussey trans.). La Salle, Illinois: Open Court.

———. 1994. *Man a Machine; and, Man a Plant* (Justin Leiber and Maya Rybalka trans.). Indianapolis: Hackett Publishing Company.

Gandhi, M. K. 1992. *Key to Health*. Ahmedabad: Navajivan Press.
Harvey, W. 1993. *The Circulation of the Blood* (Kenneth J. Franklin trans.). London: Everyman.
Sharma, P. V. (trans.). 1981. *Carakasamhita*. Varanasi: Chaukhambha Orientalia.

Nine

Network of Touch in Spiritual Healing

Panchikarana-prakriya

Piyali Palit

Living beings on earth are found to react to touch right from their birth. Even before they have visual sensation of their surroundings, they respond to sound and touch quite naturally. The reasons behind this may be found in the process of their creation. The event of creation, especially of this world, appears to be a mystery for people, leaving ample scope for speculation. In the Indian tradition, beings on this earth have always been looked upon as *amrtasya putrah* — descendants of the Eternal Being. Simultaneously, it is also believed that this being is none but that *atman*, who by nature is *sat, cit* and *ananda*; that is, eternity, knowledge and bliss are inherent qualities of all beings of this world. In the *Rgveda*, this is described as:

> हिरण्यगर्भः समवर्तताग्रे भूतस्य जातः प्रतिरेक आसीत् ।।
> (ऋग्वेदः ।१०।१२१)

viz., that *Hiranyagharbha*, the only one present prior to the creation of this world, remains the lord of all beings. In the *Taittiriya Upanisad*, we find:

> तस्मादवा एतस्मादात्मनो आकाशः सम्भूतः आाकाशदवायुः
> वायोरग्निः अग्नेरापः अन्भ्यः पृथिवीः।। तै।उ।३।१।८।

While illustrating the process of creation, Advaita Vedantins are found to quote this sentence in favour of *panchikarana-prakriya*: the five basic elements referred to in the statement above are created in a chain from 'that *atman*' or real nature of each and every being. But this *atman* is itself devoid of physique and physical attributes, with words such as *akayam*, *asnaviram*, *abranam*, *apapabiddham*, and *arogam*, all negating corporeality, used in the scriptures. That is why there is eternal bliss associated with eternal consciousness and perennial existence. Similarly, this primal entity, or Brahman, being *niravayava* (without parts), can never be the cause of creation either, since creation presupposes transformation from its existence as a whole prior to creation, or separation from its original essence, or alteration of the relations between its components, and so on. The cessation of relations between its components, admitting the absence of the *atman* itself in the form of *pragabhava,* or imbalance in its components; *samyavastha-chyuti* or *viparinama,* or the interference of some other external cause appearing to be the real cause; *vivarta,* and such other ways to account for creation, would all contradict the nature of the ultimate reality as understood in the tradition. To clear such ambiguity or confusion in the sentences describing the creation of the world, notions of *sahakari-karana* (secondary or contributory cause) as *maya* or *shakti* (illusion or power), often referred to as *kundalini* (the coiled serpent power), have been widely accepted.

However, let us now concentrate on the word *sambhuta* in the sentence referred to above. This word obviously indicates *bhava-pratyaya* — forming with *bhavati* a universal verb, meaning 'to be'. *Bhava-pratyaya,* in fact, expresses a meaning of co-location with any other properties, leading to complex structures like thing-kind, their relationships, and abstract pervasion in time and space. Most importantly, *bhava-pratyaya* necessarily implies two conditions:

- Atomic form of pervasion like manhood and humanness; and
- Punctuation between entity and its kind, for example, man || manhood, human || humanness, etc.

It is to be noted that such expressions are not propositions or sets. On the contrary, they were used as sortal tools, as a kind of abstraction device, traditionally known as *jati* or *samanya* and *visesa*, and their particular relationship as *samavaya* or relation of inherence. This principle of sortal abstraction has been explicitly illustrated by Navjyoti Singh in Vaisesika Formal Ontology, or theories of Navya Vaisesikas. In this context, he also claims that formal reasoning concerning entities in Indian tradition has been performed in two ways, 'Forms of Contiguity' and 'Forms of Pervasion'.[1] Maintaining this form of contiguity in each and every entity in this world, we find a universal principle featuring six types of *vikara*s as stated in *Nirukta*, a *vedanga* known as Vedic etymology. Yaska, the author of *Nirukta*, quotes one Varsyayani as stating:

> षड्भावविकारा भवन्ति इति वार्ष्यायणि —
> जायतेऽस्ति विपरिणमते वर्धतेऽपक्षीयते विनश्यतीति।।निरूक्त।।१।१।२
>
> All the *bhava padartha*s are found to go through six types of contiguous transformations, namely:
>
> Birth→Existence→Growth→Deformation→Decrease (and finally)→ Death or Destruction.

Here arises the contradiction: how is it that human beings, who by nature are *atman* which is *satchitananda*, are captured by six types of *vikaaras* and continuously go through *duhkha* — *adhyatmika, adhibhautika* and *adhidaivika* — arising out of their own actions? One way out of the contradiction, to quote Navjyoti Singh, is to suggest that 'Persons are clustered objectifications of Differentiating — Traces of any Self' (ibid). In defence of this statement, we may quote the Patanjala *sutra*: *sati mule tad-vipakah jatyaurbhogah* (Patanjala sutram.2.13): each and every being from their very birth acts in specific ways, accruing various but definite results. The accumulation of such deeds constructs a 'person as a social being', as well as what we really understand as 'life'. Thus, although a person does not differ from his being as Self, he simply enjoys or suffers from his own clustered objectification centring round the 'I' or '*aham*'. This happens to be the root cause of all kinds of 'dis-ease', as against the natural 'ease' which is his normal property.

If so, how to avoid disastrous or negative situations depends on our discriminative power or *viveka-buddhi*. Here, we may ask how classical Indian philosophies might help. Fundamentally, Indian philosophies offer formal insights into how suturing occurs with the form of contiguity and form of pervasion. To quote Navjyoti Singh, 'They are formal systems of punctuators and their relational context' (Singh, ibid). He presents evidence in favour of his thesis from the *Nirukta*:

> मनुष्याः कस्मात् ।मत्वा कमीणि
> सीव्यन्तीति। (निरूक्तम्३।२।१)

What is the reason behind defining a being as *manusya*? It is simply because 'they stitch their actions after mentation'. Further evidence is found in the text of Nighantu, the source-book of *Nirukta*: मनुष्याः पञ्चजनाः।। (निघण्टुः।३।२). These definitions for human beings were recorded at least in the 5th century BC, and were brought back into cognisance by Navjyoti Singh while constructing the Vaisesika formal ontology and establishing Indian forms of reasoning in describing the human being as a contiguous form in punctuation. This formal definition describes the human being as one who stitches action after mentation, which reveals his position in the network of this world as one who enjoys every freedom in building up his life or his world according to his own actions stitched with mentation.

Action for human beings, as for any being, is possible only when they acquire compatible bodies made out of the five elements mentioned in the sentence 'तस्माद् वा' — *akasha*, *vayu*, *agni*, *ap*, and *prthvi*. All five elements are the loci of five *tanmatra*s or specific *guna*s, viz., *sabda* in *akasha*, *sparsha* in *vayu*, *rupa* in *agni*, *rasa* in *ap*, and *gandha* in *prthvi*. The combination of these five assorted elements, described as *panchikarana*, evolves as different kinds of bodies — *sharira* as *bhogayatana*, where *bhoga* occurs through actions. Thus, human bodies are found to be nothing but *sanantarya* or punctuated forms of these elements, *bhuta* (physical) and *tanmatra* (transphysical) in the contiguous form of *atman* (*nairantarya*).

In this system of *panchikarana*, a causal hierarchy of the five elements along with their *guna*s or *tanmatra*s has been maintained, whereby it is found that *akasha* | | *shabda* occupies the highest order of purity and extension, followed by *vayu* | | *sparsha*, *agni* | | *rupa*, *ap* | | *rasa*, and *prthvi* | | *gandha*. The word *panca* used in this context is of utmost importance, indicating the 'Form of Contiguity' as noted by Navjyoti Singh (ibid.) while illustrating the Vaisesika formal ontology. The term *panca* derives from the root *panca*, meaning to spread, to extend, to file in, etc. When these elements remain without extension, that is, without encroaching upon one another, they are named *apancikrta*. When they extend, encroaching upon one another, they transform into *pancikrta*. As such, *parthiva-dravya*s are found to be made of 1/5th *prthvi* | | *gandha* combined with 1/4th of the other four couplets, at the maximum. Quantitative and qualitative variations in the elements are possible, and this makes the world full of variety. It is notable that all these five elements are present in each and every *dravya* having 'that *atman*' as their generator. The application of the term *panca* in this context virtually proves the 'theory of punctuator' introduced by Navjyoti Singh, which is not in contradiction with the intention of the Vaidika *rishis*. In fact, it will not be out of context to provide a brief illustration of the theory to understand the process of creation recorded in the Upanishads.

The word *panch,* with its Indo-European root, is found in other linguistic cultures too: punctum, point, punctual, puncture, expunge, punctu/punctual, disappoint, poignant. Compunctio/compunction is to be pricked by one's own sting, and usually indicates the prick of conscience. All these applications may be concorded in a single term as punctuation or punctuator (tool of punctuation). The significance of this term is 'a non-geometrical idea of point', which reveals the discreteness of each and every entity along with their relations. This point or punctuator is essentially a non-entity without which entities can never find their existence. Form of pervasion thus finds its place in this form of punctuation.

The five basic elements normally require to be punctuated to reach the form of pervasion for creation, as it has been formalised in *panchikarana-prakriya*. Hence, each and every one of the *pancha mahabhutas* is to be found in causal relation, that is, punctuated as cause | | effect, although they are able to maintain their discreteness as assorted with their specific *guna*, *karma* and *visesa*, as well as *jati* located in their *paramanas*. This form of punctuation has been shown in Figure 9.1.

Figure 9.1: Forms of Punctuation

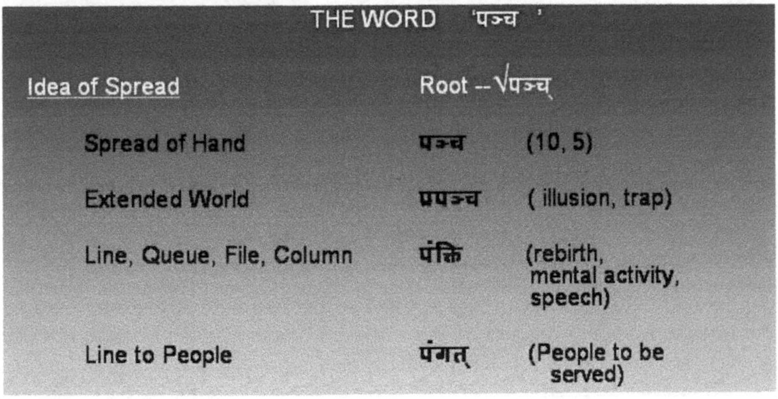
THE WORD 'पञ्च'
Idea of Spread
Root -- √पञ्च्
Spread of Hand
पञ्च
(10, 5)
Extended World
प्रपञ्च
(illusion, trap)
Line, Queue, File, Column
पंक्ति
(rebirth, mental activity, speech)
Line to People
पंगत्
(People to be served)

Needless to say, it is only this process of *panchikarana* that constitutes the quantitative and qualitative variations in the elements, this variegated world, and human bodies too. As we have already seen, following *niruktakara*, the natural course of quantitative and qualitative changes are: originating, existing, transforming, growing, degenerating and destroying forms. This should also be regarded as the universal principle of sickness and healing — two phases or aspects that everybody in this world experiences. Even vegetable and animal forms of life are not beyond this principle; indeed, no exception in this regard has been found till date. It may be argued that if sickness and healing are taken to be as part of the natural course of life, or quantitative and qualitative changes, there might not be any necessity for 'treatment' at all.

Why does one seek help to get rid of suffering or disease? The body–mind complex that renders the form of a being with consciousness at its core is felt to be the locus of all pain/pleasure, while the functional aspect of this complex presents the truth behind it. The body, or a mass enveloped with skin, cannot by itself produce the awareness of

Figure 9.2: Pancha Mahabhuta and Tanmatra Forms of Punctuation

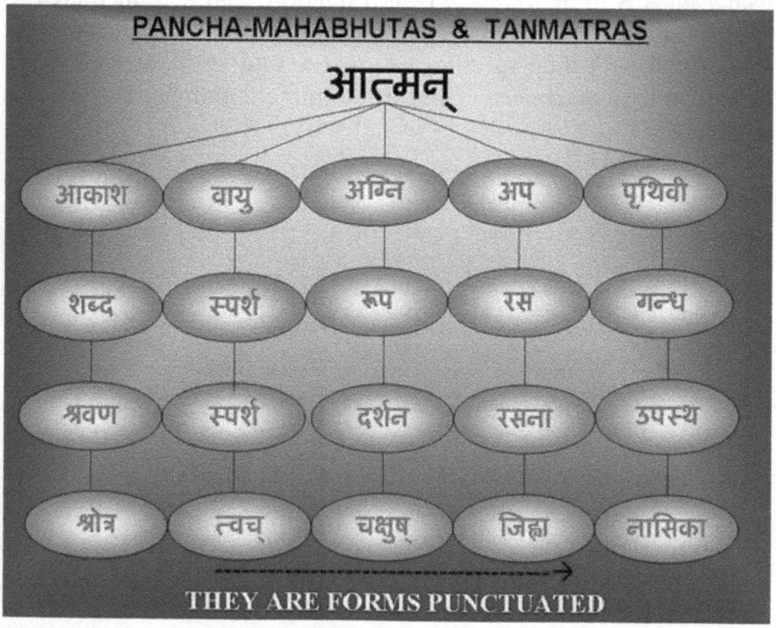

pain/pleasure unless and until the 'mind' or *antahkarana* fills the gap between the *jada* (non-conscious) body and *cit* (conscious) *atman*; that is how we become aware of such conditions as pain/pleasure, felt as caused through contact with external entities. Contact with external entities is channelised through the sense organs, while awareness of sensation finds its place only in the *atman*. We are marked by disease only when we restrict our pain/pleasure either to our physical body or to our mind and detach ourselves from our *atman*, which is beyond the principle of qualitative or quantitative changes, the *bhava-vikaras*. However, because pain/pleasure is reality for us, it requires all possible kinds of treatment, whether physical and mental.

Touch or *sparsha*, the most pervasive quality associated with *vayu*, is found to be capable of treating the body and mind so as to bring them back to ease from disease. What is meant by 'touch'? Touch may be translated simply as *tvaca-pratyaksa* or tactile perception. *Tvaca-pratyaksa* is a cognitive state produced by a series of entities in relation, where *vayu* plays the main role. *Tvagindriya*/tactile organ, a *karmendriya* as well as a *jnanendriya* known as *sparshendriya* are products of a particular *tanmatra*—*sparsha*, which is again basically associated with *vayu*. At the same time, our skin is made not only of *vayu*, but also of a transformation of all the other elements pervaded and mixed up in certain portions lower than *vayu*. Hence, when a mass-form enveloped with skin comes into contact or *samsarga* with another mass-form enveloped with skin, we call it 'touch', through which we practically get into touch/contact with other elements. In the case of healing, impurity in the body is thus supposed to be eliminated and/or replaced by pure elements through channels existing in punctuated forms. At the same time, another set of entities known as *panca-prana*, having their special forms purely out of *vayu*, function to ease the mental state. According to Vaishesikas, the mind, a transformed state of *manas*, having the quantity of a *paramanu* as well as the quality of subtleness and void of consciousness, that is, *jada* and *suksma*, waits for *vayu* to activate it. The movement of *vayu* inside the body helps the mind to make us feel pain/pleasure. Advaita Vedantins, however, regard the mind as *antahkarana*, understood to be a transformation of *tejas*/*agni*, only unlike other *bhauta dravya*s. The *antahkarana* is nothing but a transparent stretchable form of *tejas* acting as a link between matter (including both *indriyas* and external objects) and *atman*. Therefore, the sensation of touch occurs with the help of the *antahkarana* stretching, transferring that sensation to the *atman* of a being. The stretching of the *antahkarana*, known as *antahkarana-vrtti*, occurs in assistance with *prana-vayu*. While healing through touch, thus, *vayu* occupies the largest extension over our body and mind, that is, *bhautika-sharira*, affecting the balance mechanism in association with the other four elements in proper combination. Any imbalance in this mechanism causes stress upon the total system, leading to what we call 'disease'. So, whenever one thinks of 'healing' or treatment of any kind of disease, this bundle of totality should be kept in mind.

The most important question for a healer as it stands now is: What is healing? From the perspective of *panchikarana*, healing should be looked upon as the replacement of degenerated parts by freshly generated ones. Generation afresh can be initiated by the manual touch of the healer, in which energy radiation becomes possible through channels and points in the skin of the person to be healed. Energy radiation as a curative method is very much possible, and often found to happen even if the healer and the healed are not in direct physical touch. *Vayu*, being the most pervasive element next to *akasha*, invariably makes each and every body in touch with one another, whether we are aware of it or not. Naturally, we experience many things in terms of pain/pleasure without knowing well the underlying causes of such experiences. When touch-healing is done with full awareness of the total system, it is noted as *yoga*, that is, being related. The process of *yoga* or being related affects the mind since it is effectuated by the *citta*, a form of *manas*, with the help of *prana*, a special form of *vayu*.

This traditional process of treatment is in practice among the Advaita Vedantins with the objective of healing the fundamental disease caused by *avidya*, that is, not knowing one's own self because of the adverse situation of being in *sanantarya* or form punctuated. A common practice of theirs is that while meditating, they focus on the basic elements and their causal role in maintaining the body, and dissolve them in reverse method to reach the core state of *Brahma-chaitanya* or awareness of one's own infinitude.

Touch-Healing Applied in Modern Practice

Quantum-Touch is one of the modern, popular practices of healing through touch. It is an energy healing modality that applies the principles of resonance or vibration and entrainment to facilitate healing. It is also known as Vibration Therapy. Vibration is created by raising the *kundalini shakti* lying dormant in every body. Through the practice of *Raja yoga*, *shakti* or life-force can be raised up to the *sahasrara* through six *granthis* or *sthanas* located in the body in alignment with the *meru-danda* or backbone. In the introduction to this chapter, a reference was made to *kundalini* while explaining the process of cosmic creation. The human body, being a replica of the universe, follows the universal principle of qualitative and quantitative changes as observed by the Vaidika *rishis*. In this process, as illustrated in Patanjala-darshana or Yoga philosophy, practitioners learn to focus and *amplify* life-force energy, or *prana* ('*Chi*' in Chinese), by combining various breathing and body-awareness exercises known as *pranayam* in the process of practising *Raja yoga*. When the practitioner resonates at a high frequency, the client often entrains to, or matches, the higher frequency, thereby facilitating healing using the body's biological intelligence, as described by the modern practitioners.

To conclude, life-force energy affects matter on the quantum, sub-atomic level, and works its way up through atoms, molecules, cells, tissues, and structure. To make life-force energy affect matter on the quantum level, all the points or punctuators must be made to be in touch in a series with the help of the *antahkarana* associated with *prana*. This is what *panchakarana* actually does. The sensation of touch or vibration occurs with the help of the *antahkarana* stretching, transferring that sensation to the *atman* of a being. While healing through touch, thus, one can touch even one's inner self. Moreover, by the recursive method involved, one can eliminate the basic impurities deposited through one's action and open the door to purity. Expressed in the form of *aum*, the divine in sound aids this process of healing. The practice of *pranayam* is thus essentially associated with *aum-kaara-upasana*, as prescribed in all the traditional texts.

Note

1. Singh's work is widely known in the field, but scarcely available; see Tavva and Singh (2010) for an example of his approach.

Reference

Tavva, Rajesh and Navjyoti Singh. 2010. 'Generative Graph Grammar of Neo-Vaiśeṣika Formal Ontology (NVFO)', in G.N. Jha (ed.), *Sanskrit Computational Linguistics*, LNCS 6465, pp. 91–105, http://www.academia.edu/904198/Generative_Graph_Grammar_of_Neo-Vaise_ika_Formal_Ontology_NVFO (accessed 3 March 2014).

Ten

Bio-ethical Issues

Jaina Perspective and Prospects

Asha Mukherjee

During the past two centuries, the West has experienced dramatic developments in science and technology, especially in the bio-sciences. This has changed the life pattern of human beings and has affected the planet tremendously. But science does not happen in a vacuum; it is either supported or restricted by the society and culture in which it functions. Each culture and society has its own 'science', and the interaction between science and society has its own norms. Science in the Asian context has its own logic, methodology, and epistemology as it is practised. This may lead to a clash or uneasy co-existence between what we call 'traditional' science and modern, or the so-called 'universal', science. Pre-modern science and modern science may simply be seen as alternative knowledge systems. Keeping this mode of understanding of science, in this chapter we concentrate on the issues related with bio-ethics from a Jaina perspective, which is one of the major Asian philosophical traditions. Religions do not remain static, and perhaps through the Jaina perspective we can see the emergence of a modern ethical discourse within and for a laity, whose concerns throughout history has generally been more diverse and variable than those of the ascetic community.

Bio-ethics refers to a 'new discipline that combines biological knowledge with a knowledge of the human value system' (Potter 1975: 2299), bridging the gap between science, medical science and humanities, helping humanities to survive, and sustain and improve the civilised world. It encompasses issues related with healthcare, confidentiality, honesty, autonomy for children; life and death issues, such as abortion, the moral status of the human embryo, foetus, new-born, etc., allowing patients to die, brain-dead patients, permanently unconscious patients in a vegetative state; the meaning of recovery and the interests of the individual as a patient vs. the interests of 'others'; the distribution of resources to healthcare as a social and organisational need; fair distribution, and who gets to decide what is fair; issues related to 'new genetics', organ transplantation, prolonging the 'natural' life of human beings and animals through medicine and surgery; affecting and interfering with the 'natural order' — test-tube babies, cloning, sex-change operations, etc. The moral status of all sentient living beings, including plants, fall within the scope of ethical concern.

I propose to work out the response to these issues, which arose mainly from 1970 onwards due to modern scientific and medical advancements, from the Jaina perspective. This response will be worked out from Jaina logic, methodology and epistemology. This involves a basic understanding of the Jaina view of God, the universe, creation, obligations of laymen and ascetics, the theory of *karma*, freedom of human beings, obligation towards oneself and towards the universe as a whole, and the basic principle of *ahimsa*, which is extremely important in understanding the Jaina perspective.

Most of the moral concepts vital for bio-ethics — autonomy, self-rule, the ability to make decisions for oneself on the basis of deliberation and self-determination, acting in a way that benefits others, treating people equally and providing justice in relation to their needs, rights, merits and demerits, and abilities, not harming others, owing other people the highest level of moral respect — are all discussed in the Jaina philosophical system. Who is to be regarded as an 'individual' is a matter of debate in the scheme of bio-ethics, but not in Jaina philosophy. Whether human embryos, foetuses, newborn babies, and permanently unconscious and brain-dead patients surviving on ventilators can be regarded as 'individuals' is a contested area in bio-ethics; however, Jaina philosophy has a clear position on this.

From the Jaina perspective, all are given the status of individuals, which, as I argue, follows from their theory of *karma*, their worldview, and their law of *ahimsa*. We may agree on the universal obligation to refraining from unjustly killing each other; who, though, is the 'other' within the Jaina framework? We may agree that we have an obligation to respect other people's autonomy, but who can be counted as 'autonomous'? To what extent do we have 'autonomous' agents in the Jaina framework? We may agree on the principle of distributive justice, but how do we distribute the resources justly, and among whom? These are the questions we need to address within the Jaina framework, and there may not be easy answers.

Jainism is among the most modern and scientific ancient philosophies, where the principles of equality and freedom are recognised to promote welfare. The two basic tenets of Jainism are *anekantavada* and *ahimsa*: the principles of peaceful co-existence, both philosophically and socially. Our problems with bio-ethics have to be addressed from these perspectives. *Ahimsa* is accepted as the regulative principle of conduct in practical life, as well as the spiritual path and a guiding principle for our outlook and thought. *Ahimsa* is the principle of respect for life and *anekanta* is the doctrine of open-mindedness. *Ahimsa* recognises equality in all beings and completely rejects the idea of domination over the other. *Anekanta* is the principle that urges the comprehension of a thing from different points of view. *Anekantavada*, along with its corollaries — *nayavada* and *syadvada* — provides the basis for different kinds of integration and intellectual respect for each other. In Jaina epistemology, we find that *samyak caritra* (right conduct) has been given more importance than knowledge.

Jainism uses a dialectical method to address every issue, whether spiritual or practical. In this chapter, we will try to address the problems of bio-ethics by using the dialectical method employed by Jainism, and understand their logical implications.

Jaina Philosophical Perspective and its Identity

In Jaina philosophy, great sanctity is attached to all life. The soul is taken as a conscious substance. The word 'Jaina' means a conqueror, who has obtained perfect knowledge and absolute freedom from the bondage of *karma*. It refers especially to the *tirthankara,* the one who has built a passage through the ocean of births, that is, the teachers of this religion. Sometimes *tirthankara* is also understood to mean the founder of the four *tirtha*s, or the orders of the monks and the nuns. Twenty-four *tirthankara*s had conquered their passion and sought liberation, of whom Rsabha or Adinath was the first. Historically, only the existence of Mahavira is traceable, and that of Parsvanatha may be inferred. The essential teachings were canonised only in the 3rd century BC, and were recorded in written form several centuries later. Bihar was the main centre of Mahavira's followers, but after a famine in the region, a large group of monks left Bihar and migrated to Karnataka. One group, however, stayed back in Magadh. The ones who migrated and stuck to the strict regulations became known as *digambara*, 'the sky-robed', while the latter who stayed back, and changed their ways due to the famine, became known as *svetambara* or 'white-robed'. The *svetambara* are further divided into two sub-sects, namely *deravasi* — those who worship the idol in a temple — and *sthanakvasi* — those who worship their teachers in a monastery. The *digambaras* were divided into *terapanthi* and *bisapanthi*, depending on differences in ritual observance. Jainism found patronage in early rulers like Chandragupta Maurya, Ashoka, Kharvela of Kalinga, etc. In order to avoid injury to living organisms, agriculture and animal husbandry were prohibited in Jainism. Occupations involving less mobility, such as those of merchants, were more suitable. This is why Jainas chose as their preferred occupation the owning of large businesses such as textile industries, chemical industries, newspapers, precious metals, jewellery, and banking.

Jainas realise that a strict moral discipline is necessary for the purity of life. They do not isolate metaphysics from the nature of the self; behaviour cannot be isolated from our metaphysical beliefs. Truth and value are inseparable; without knowing the truth, values cannot be realised — and that is the ultimate aim of philosophy. Therefore, metaphysics and ethics are two sides of the same coin. Samantabhadra goes to the extent of saying that without knowing the real nature of things, which is permanency in transience, all moral distinctions between bondage and liberation, *papa* and *punya*, heaven and hell, pleasure and pain will be blurred (Bhargava 1968: 12). *Nayavada* represents the most consistent and logical form of realism in Indian metaphysics. *Syadvada* constitutes a comprehensive scheme of complementary methods designed to help the mind to grasp the nature of reality, in its unity as well as its diversity. All evil traits of character arising out of speech, mind or body have to be eradicated before the attainment of final emancipation.

Every object known to us has innumerable characteristics, besides positive and negative implications of what it is and what it is not. The set of what it is not will always be greater than what it is, which also changes with time. Whatever the nature of the object, it is due to its *gunas* (substantial qualities). There could also be accidental qualities. Consciousness is a substantial quality of the soul, but pleasure, pain and desire are accidental (modes or *paryayas*) to soul-substance. Both change and permanence are real. Reality consists of three factors: permanence, origination and decay. Souls have varying degrees and kinds of knowledge. There could be perfect souls who have attained omniscience, or there could be low and still lower varieties of imperfect souls, which inhabit bodies in earth, water, air, or vegetables. Two to five-sensed are midway between the lowest and highest; examples of these include worms, ants, and also men. The soul is eternal, but it undergoes a change of state. On the basis of one's past actions, a *jiva* enters a body. *Jiva* is not infinite; it is not present everywhere, but only in the body. Jainas reject the existence of God as the creator of the world, but the notion of worship is well-accepted in the system. One should worship the liberated or perfect souls, they are God-like and can be prayed to; they can offer guidance and provide inspiration. Past misdeeds can only be countered by generating strong opposite forces like good thought, good speech, and good action within the soul. Therefore, everyone must work towards his own salvation.

Jainism accepts the dualism between self and non-self — *jiva*, the soul, and *ajiva*, the matter. How the *jiva* joins *ajiva* is a mystery, but it is *karmic* matter that is the medium between body and soul. The soul has an inherent quality that attracts these particles towards itself. But the mere flow of this *karmic* matter is not an obstacle in itself; rather, it is in combination with the four fundamental passions — anger, pride, deceitfulness, and greed — that the *karmic* matter is held in bondage with the soul. This inflow of fresh *karmic* matter is to be (*samvara*) checked. This requires constant vigilance against those trends of mind, deeds and words that may lead to such inflow. One needs to shed *karmic* matter, already accumulated by the soul, with the help of meditation. In the end, the soul that was engulfed in the mud of *karmic* matter shines in its intrinsic purity of infinite knowledge, intuition, bliss, and potency (Umasvati 2002: 1.4).

The attainment of right conduct is a gradual process; the aspirant may not be able to achieve the highest ideals at the first stage. He can therefore observe only partial self-control as a householder, whereas at the stage of monkhood, he becomes capable of observing the rules of conduct more extensively. So we have two sets of rules of conduct — one for householders and another for monks.

The roles of our intellect, effort, and moral teachings as helpers (teachers) are only meaningful if freedom of will is accepted. It makes no sense to tell a person who has no choice what he should or should not do. The theory of omniscience and the theory of *karma* do presuppose a kind of determinism, but do not come in the way of our efforts to make ourselves moral. Kundakunda says that all of us have a two-fold consciousness: *jnanacetana* or knowledge consciousness, and *karmacetana* or action consciousness (Bhargava 1968: 33), thereby bestowing upon us a kind of freedom of will.

Knowledge consciousness refers to the state of absolute freedom from the sense of being the agent of an action. The soul remains in its pure, intrinsic, blissful, conscious state. It has no desire to initiate action and is in a supra-moral state, beyond good or bad — the state of complete freedom. But from a practical point of view, it is action consciousness that dominates one's activities. Man has to choose between the conflicting emotions of good and evil. It is here that the role of the *purusarthas* (human effort) comes in. The two consciousnesses exclude each other and cannot exist side by side. The road to a supra-ethical plane of life is only through the practical path of morality, and not through immorality. The ultimate aim is complete cessation of all activities and attainment of knowledge consciousness. But it is only the self's effort and exertion that brings it closer to its goal. The self, within self, satisfied with only the self — the motto of all individualistic systems of philosophy — is a kind of inwardness. In general, Indian systems accept that extroversion, whether due to our incapability for self-control or for the cause of social service, never leads us closer to the goal of spiritual attainment. Rather, it is withdrawal from the outside world which takes us closer to self-realisation.

The bondage of a soul is associated with matter, so it must disassociate itself from matter by *stopping* the influx of new matter into the soul and completely eliminating the matter with which the soul is mixed up. These two methods are called *samvara* and *nirjara*. To remove ignorance, one must have the right knowledge. Mere knowledge is useless in itself; it must be practised through right conduct. Through *samvara* and *nirjara*, a soul is liberated by eliminating matter which enmeshes the soul in bondage. Liberation from this bondage is the joint effect of three gems: right faith (respect for truth), right knowledge, and right conduct.

To ascertain correct knowledge, one has to make personal effort. A practical code of conduct has been provided in this system. Vows compulsory for Jainas are *ahimsa* (abstinence from all injury to life), *satyam* (abstaining from falsehood), and *brahamcharya* (abstinence from self-indulgence). In total, there are five vows for any Jaina: *satyam, ahimsa, astayam, brahamcharya*, and *aparigraha*.

Parigraha is the result of *mohakarma*, the main obstacle to self-realisation. *Moha* has two sides: attachment and aversion. The first manifests itself as *parigraha* and the second as *himsa*. Therefore, *aparighraha* is as important as *ahimsa*; it is non-attachment as well as non-possession. *Parigraha* includes land, house, coins, gold, servants, jewels, beds, and other items of luxury. There are some other vows for householders, known as *silavratas*. These include three *gunavratas* and four *siksavratas* — like restricting the movement of a householder in order to avoid violence (Bhargava 1968: 128).

The Jainas believe that a soul takes residence in a new body after the death of its present one according to its volitional activities. This is accomplished by the soul drawing towards itself a subtle kind of matter or *karman*, which then envelops it and defines the new body it will receive. If the soul becomes subject to attachment and aversion, it becomes harmful (*himsa*), both to itself and to others. If, instead, it maintains detachment and compassion, the soul comes to be non-injurious (*ahimsa*) towards all beings. The Jaina thus defines *himsa* as something ultimately linked to one's personal mental state, involving injury primarily to oneself. *Ahimsa*, and the awareness of *ahimsa*, becomes a constant concern for the individual, involving total mindfulness in mental, oral, and physical activities. The orientation of the Jaina discussion on *ahimsa* thus proceeds from the perspective of one's own soul, and is not so much about the protection of other beings or the welfare of humanity as a whole. *Ahimsa* is therefore a creed in its own right: identified with one's own spiritual impulses and informing all of one's activities, it may truly be termed a way towards personal discipline.

The social implication of what is fundamentally a personal salvation enterprise can be found in Jaina texts. There are two explicit schemes of vows, called *anuvrata* (minor vows) and *mahavratas* (major vows), applicable to lay people and monks, respectively. Jaina monks are known for life-long vows of renunciation of all worldly possessions and all acts of violence in any form, towards both humans and animals. The monks were the embodiments of *ahimsa*. Three different kinds of *himsa* can be expressed. True *ahimsa* means not only refraining from inflicting injury on others, but also renouncing the very will towards the attachment and aversion that initiates such violence. *Samkalpaja himsa* (harm intentionally planned and carried out) or wilful violence, and *arambhja-himsa* (occupational violence) are to be minimised or renounced altogether. The larger questions facing modern society, such as national defence, weapons of mass destruction, limiting the population of wild animals and insect-pests, the use of toxic chemicals, the morality of capital punishment, the use of animals in medical research, and other social concerns that entail violence were beyond the pale of Jaina thought.

Jainas extended their dietary restrictions to various types of vegetable life as well. In their attempts to categorise those types of plants that could be consumed with relatively less harm, the Jaina developed a whole science of botany that was rather unique in Indian religious history. For example, eating fruits and vegetables containing a large number of seeds (*bahubija*), such as figs or eggplants, was not favoured; single-stone fruits like mangoes attracted no restrictions. Jainas recognised that plants were the lowest form of life since they possessed only a single sense, that of touch; they could be eaten, provided they are harvested and prepared with care. Thus, vegetarianism is prescribed to develop positive mental states that will ultimately be to an individual's personal benefit. Mahavira says,

> [n]o being in the world is to be harmed by a spiritually inclined person whether knowingly or unknowingly, for all beings desire to live and no being wishes to die. A true Jaina therefore, consciously refrains from harming any being, however small (Lalvani 1973: 11).

For laymen, just war and violence in defence of one's property, honour, family, community, or nation were not so explicitly characterised. In these matters, the individual had to take into account not only his duties to himself, but also those towards society as a whole. The duty of a monk, in this case, was quite clear; he must not retaliate in any way and must be willing to lay down his own life in order to keep his vow of total non-violence. For laymen, there were always situations in which violence could be a last resort to guard his own and his community's interests. Thus *virodhi himsa*, or counter-violence, could be justified, albeit as a final resort. Even mercy killing is a form of violence (*Purusarthasiddhyupaya* 85). The suffering animal is a victim of his own past *karmanas*, and his suffering cannot be cut short by killing him (Bhargava 1968: 114).

In upholding that one may have complete control over one's own destiny by arranging the conditions prevalent at one's death, the Jainas have even gone as far as proclaiming that abandoning one's own life in a controlled manner is a legitimate act. As Padmanabh S. Jaini has noted in his *Collected Papers on Jaina Studies* (2000), this was known, technically, as *sallekhana*. The word literally means 'thinning one's own body and passions', and implies a 'ritualized form of self-killing allowed only to monks, nuns, and under special circumstances to advanced laypersons' (ibid.: 16). As Professor Jaini notes, however, several conditions govern the act of *sallekhana*. First, it can only be undertaken by public declaration, and never in private. Second, death may only be brought about by gradually withdrawing from the consumption of any food or water. Also, it is to be noted that one is forbidden from beginning such a fast until death is a certainty, and is imminent; a fact that has to be verified by teachers and colleagues of the person who is dying. Thus, the only situation or condition in which a request by a monk to begin s*allekhana* would be granted by his superiors would be one where total disability or terminal illness have been preventing him from keeping his vows. 'The basic justification for *sallekhana*', Jaini explains, 'is that a person who has conscientiously led a holy life has earned the right to die in peace in full possession of his faculties, without any attachment to worldly bonds, including his own body' (Jaini 2000: 16). The person must first admit to the transgression of the moral vows made earlier. Desiring to neither artificially lengthen life nor unduly anticipate his demise, the individual thus allows his life to ebb away naturally, while still in complete possession of his faculties.

According to Jainas, every judgement is to be qualified by a word like *shayad* (maybe). Truth is manifold and to make a categorical judgement is to claim that it is only of one kind, which is not only wrong, but also dogmatic. Every judgement only expresses one aspect of reality, and is therefore relative to conditions. Different systems of philosophy present partial aspects of reality. The Jaina system insists that we should always use a qualifier to express our view. For example, instead of saying 'It is raining', one should say, 'Maybe it is raining'. This indicates the space, time, quality, etc., under which it is raining. This way of making judgements avoids the possibility of misunderstanding that it is raining at all times and everywhere. It emphasises that ordinary judgements passed by imperfect minds hold good from particular aspects, in particular circumstances, and from that point of view.

The earliest known text, *Acaranga Sutra*, lists the different forms of life in detail and advocates various techniques for their protection. The text states: 'All breathing, existing, living, sentient creatures should not be slain, nor treated with violence, nor abused, or tormented, nor driven away. This is pure, unchangeable, eternal law' (1989: Book 1, Lecture 4, Lesson 1). The *Acaranga Sutra* talks about avoiding harm not only to animals, but also to plants, by not touching them, and to the bodies that dwell on earth, water, fire, and air. According to the *Tattvarthasutra*, there are 8,400,000 different species of life forms. These beings are part of a ceaseless round of birth, life, death, and rebirth. Each living being houses a life force or *jiva* that occupies and enlivens the host environment. When the body dies, the *jiva* seeks out a new site, depending on the proclivities of karma generated and accrued during the previous lifetime. Depending upon one's action, one can either ascend to a heavenly realm and be reborn as a human or animal or elemental form, or descend into one of the hells as a suffering human being or a particular animal. Although the resultant lifestyles for monks and nuns resemble or approximate an environmentally friendly ideal, its pursuits focus on personal spiritual advancement, not on a holistic vision of the interrelatedness of life. In terms of the lifestyle of the Jaina lay person, certain practices such as vegetarianism, periodic fasting, and eschewal of militarism might be seen as eco-friendly.

According to Jainism, time, space, life, and non-life (matter) exist and will exist forever. Life in the universe is mainly regulated by *karmas*, unless these are all removed through a prescribed path of purification. This is not easy, since Jainism believes in existing *karmic* matter, which can only be removed (before a predetermined duration) through austerity; otherwise, the personal *karmic* computer will continue working. It prescribes self-restraint rather than self-indulgence. The bondage of the soul is associated with matter, and so must disassociate itself from matter by the two methods of *samvara* and *nirjara* (discussed earlier).

Important Contributions of Jaina Philosophy

First, it provides space for a difference of opinion and avoids any absolutist stand or conflict. Jainism is accepting of a kind of relativism, but not of scepticism. Jainism's approach towards an opponent is constructive, not destructive. It balances between opposites: practical and transcendental, fate and human effort, substantial cause and instrumental cause, absolute and relative, etc. Jainism argues that our knowledge in the material world is limited. One needs to realise that one's view does not represent the whole truth about anything, and therefore we must learn to appreciate and respect the other's point of view.

Second, in Jainism *moksasastra*, or the science of spirituality, is not confused with *dharmasastra* or the science of righteousness. *Dharma* is different from non-essential beliefs, which change with time and place. Social problems and welfare of the society should not be confused with the essential problem of ethics, which is emancipation.

Third, it lays emphasis on the unity of faith, knowledge and conduct. Jainism is not merely a system of certain codes of morality, but a religion to be lived in practice. Both householders and monks have to practice the rules of conduct in their lives. It is neither mere speculative philosophy nor a religion of rituals, but a comprehensive system of religion and morality as well as of thought and conduct.

Fourth, it is the life of a monk that occupies central place, as the ultimate aim of life is liberation. Thus, a complete renunciation of mundane life and embracing ascetic virtues are the merits of a higher order for Jaina *acarya*s.

Fifth, Jainism is based on diversities as well as equality of life. All souls are equal, so man, animals, insects, and plant life are all given equal importance while observing *ahimsa*. Jainism does not accept any distinction based on caste, creed or colour.

Jaina logic

The three basic tenets of Jainism are (*a*) *Anekantavada*, (*b*) *Nayavada* and (*c*) *Syadavada*. These are integral parts of the conceptual framework of Jaina philosophy. Jaina philosophy asserts that the ultimate reality has many aspects and can neither be limited to one thing or another, nor can be grasped in its completeness through any ordinary source of knowledge. This view is known as *anekantavada*. The theory of *anekantavada* is based on the multifaceted nature of reality, and insists on the correlativity of assertion and negation. Whatever is real necessarily admits of multiple characterisations in terms of an infinite number of modes or *anantadharmatmaka vastuh*. This theory is basically ontological, in the sense that it is about reality. A complete grasp of the true nature of reality requires comprehending each one of its aspects or modes. Only an infinite intellect can grasp an infinite number of modes. Ordinary human beings, having only a limited intellect, cannot completely grasp reality. This implies that all our ordinary cognitive claims about reality, expressed in judgemental forms, are tied to a particular viewpoint. *Naya* is the cognitive attitude or *abhipraya* (epistemic intention) of the knower to focus on one aspect of reality without losing sight of the fact that there are other, equally important, aspects as well. This is the logical transitional link between *anekantavada* and *nayavada*.

Now, if each ordinary cognitive judgement about reality is tied to a viewpoint and is only about some particular mode or aspect of reality, then to claim that reality is characterised exclusively by that particular mode is to make a false claim. The analogy of the blind men and the elephant applies here. The blind man who feels the elephant's leg thinks it is a pillar; the one who feels the tail deems it a rope; the one who comes in contact with the elephant's body considers it a wall; and so on. The one who has really seen an elephant knows that there is nothing to quarrel about. Each blind man's judgement expresses a partial truth, but to make such judgements absolute and exclusive by saying, 'an elephant is like a pillar and nothing else' — to claim that the judgement is true without qualification — is to turn the original true judgement into a false one. In order to preserve the element of truth, each judgement should have been asserted in a qualified manner, conditionally asserted by prefixing *syat* to each: *syatgajah stambhabat eva* (conditionally speaking, an elephant is like a pillar, etc). Thus, starting from *anekantavada*, we logically reach *syadvada* via *nayavada*. It is also clear that *syadavada* is concerned with an appropriate judgemental mode of expression, with linguistic expressions.[1]

Let us look at some of the problems we face when it comes to giving a consistent interpretation of the three tenets we have discussed. According to Jainas, the real is characterised as both *sattva* (real) and *asattva* (unreal), *nitya* (eternal) and *anitya* (non-eternal), simultaneously.

How can one and the same thing possess an infinite number of properties (*dharmah*), including apparently inconsistent pairs like *sattvasattva* (existence–non-existence)? Jainas answer this question by saying that apparently inconsistent pairs like 'existence–non-existence', 'eternal–non-eternal', etc., simultaneously characterise one and the same thing only relative to different *avacchedaka*s, which is sometimes translated as 'limiters'. Pot exists *qua* a pot, but it does not exist *qua* a piece of cloth: *ghatatvene ghatah asti patatvena na*. Potness must be absent in a cloth. Potness is the class exclusion of the *dharmah*, or properties of cloth. In other words, all properties are relational properties, like 'to the left of', 'smaller than', etc., and consequently 'S is P' can significantly assert only a relative truth to a specific context.

We will not go into the details of the Jaina theory of language, but simply state the fact that all possible conditional judgements about reality can be exhaustively classified under seven possible forms of linguistic expression.[2] This is called the seven-fold scheme of *naya* or *saptabhanginaya*. Although there is an infinite number of epistemic points of view or *naya*s, all of them come under one or the other alternative in the seven-fold scheme of classification. So there are exactly seven non-overlapping and mutually exhaustive forms of *bhangas*. They are:

(a) Conditionally speaking, the pot does exist,
(b) Conditionally speaking, the pot does not exist,
(c) Conditionally speaking, the pot exists and does not exist,
(d) Conditionally speaking, the pot is indescribable,
(e) Conditionally speaking, it is indescribable, and exists,
(f) Conditionally speaking, it is indescribable, and does not exist,
(g) Conditionally speaking, it is indescribable, exists and also does not exist.

These seven *bhangas* are due to the realistic interpretation of allowing the real possibility of S's being characterised by P, or by P-complement, or by both of them together. Any one of these three modes of S's being characterised may either be linguistically expressible or linguistically inexpressible, generating thereby six *bhangas* or alternatives; three each on either side of *avaktavya*, that is, inexpressibility. Further, according to the stand taken towards the ontological state corresponding to S's mode being characterised, such that it becomes *avaktavya*, that S is neither P-characterised nor not-P characterised, is accepted in Jainism. 'Thus we may say that 'neither A nor not-A' is not even accepted as a possibility in Jainism' (Matilal 1981: 49).[3]

Moral and Social Implications

Although Jainism was originally a religious movement, it can be regarded as the first example of secularism, as it tells us that each point of view has some truth and we must respect that truth; by extension, that each religion has one perspective out of many, and we must respect each perspective. It is an example of a truly secular religion based on equal respect for all religions, and not an equal neglect of all religions. The doctrines of the manifold nature of truth and non-absoluteness provide the foundation for non-violence, which helps in overcoming religious conflict.

Jaina *dharma* originated purely from a prior consideration of both human and social needs — fellow feeling and equality on which *ahimsa* is based, the equality of all *jiva*. It is fundamentally a humanistic approach.

On the basis of Jaina principles of equality, non-violence, consequentialism, responsibility, and the principle of reciprocity, one can develop a Jaina environmental ethics.

By following Jaina principles and practising its restrictions on diet and modalities of taking food, one can regulate both mind and body, and lead a healthy and balanced life.

Jainism's non-theistic, humanitarian outlook can help to remove religious intolerance and develop a true spirit of mutual respect, tolerance and religious catholicity by reconciling various conflicting viewpoints, for instance, monotheism/polytheism, idolatry/anti-idolatry, the caste system, etc.

The Doctrine of Karma: Karma and Bio-ethics

Jaina philosophy rejects the doctrine of *karma* as put forth by most Brahmanical schools of philosophy. From the Jaina dialectical point of view, *karma* is conceived from a different perspective as belonging to the agent and not belonging to the agent: for example, all living beings, from the one-sensed to the five-sensed, are liable to sin in their actions, whether voluntary or involuntary. The philosophy accepts *kriyavada*, in the sense that suffering is caused by one's own actions, but not by the action of others. The *jiva* is confined and involved in the cycle of *karma*, which is a mark of impurity, and when the *jiva* attains liberation from the two *avaranas*, it becomes pure. Pure consciousness cannot be perceived by one's sense organs, it can only be presupposed (*arthapatti*). A *jiva* is both *karta* (actor) and *bhokta* (enjoyer); it is deeply involved in mundane affairs and is responsible for its deeds. It undergoes rebirth by virtue of its own *karma* in different realms of *samsara* until it finally attains liberation. This explanation of the doctrine of *karma* enables Jainas to establish, on the one hand, the reality of all actions in mundane affairs, and on the other, the necessary detachment for spirituality through the application of the dialectical method.

The following sections of the *Sarvartha-siddhi* deal with the theme of *karma*:

- We find, in 6.12: 'Causing pain, grief, agony, crying, injury or lamenting in oneself, or others or both, attracts pain *karma*' (Devanandi 1955: 6.12). When performing surgery, the doctor may inflict pain on the patient. But this inflicted pain does not cause an inflow of evil. Similarly, an ascetic will practice austerities that will put his body through pain. But behind such austerities is the desire to eliminate *karma* and attain liberation (Umasvati 2002: 156).

- (SS 6.12): 'Compassion through charity for all living beings, especially those observing religious vows, self restraint of a person with attachment and the like, blameless activity, forbearance, and purity (freedom from greed) cause the inflow of pleasure *karma*' (Devanandi 1955). Self-restraint, therefore, is also important in generating inflows of pleasure-producing *karma*. If both greed and self-restraint are present in equal measure, such as when a person lives his life by small (lay) vows, the power of the pleasure-producing inflow is diminished. The inflow of pleasure-producing *karma* can be attributed solely to compassion for living things, by desisting from inflicting pain. *Tattvartha Sutra* extends this description of compassion to include positive acts of charity, and also adds further factors like self-restraint as causes of the inflow of pleasure-producing karma (Umasvati 2002: 156).
- (SS 6.16): 'Deceitfulness leads to birth in animal realm' (Devanandi 1955).
- (SS 6.18): 'Attenuated aggression, attenuated possessiveness, and a soft-hearted and straightforward nature lead to birth in the human realm' (ibid.).
- (SS 6.19): 'Amorality and self-indulgence are the common cause of birth in all realms mentioned above (infernal, sub-human and human)' (ibid.).

Keeping these observations on *karma* in mind, let us turn our thoughts to the modern, scientific context of bio-ethics. Modern scientists have started cloning animals, and it is possible to clone human beings as well. We can clone whatever we want and develop any race with genes of our choice. What is the response to this from the Jaina point of view? There will be some self in the living being that is cloned, but which self would reside in which genes? That is not in the hands of scientists; science cannot determine it, but it can clone living beings with certain qualities. Science tells us that in those living beings that do not have minds, individual cells work as knowledge-collectors. How will the Jaina system respond to these scientific discoveries? Would the doctrine of *karma* as developed by Jainas be proved false? In my opinion (although, as far as I know, this problem was never specifically addressed in the Jaina texts), we can respond to this question through the philosophical underpinnings of the Jaina doctrine of *karma*. The sufferings of these cloned lives are not caused by others, but by their own activities. The *jiva* present in the cloned being is bound by its own *karma*s and is free in the realm of *samsara* until it finally attains liberation. Manipulation is a crime against the idea that there is a natural order or structure, which is perhaps divine.

In this sense, any life-saving medical treatment would also be judged by the same token. But this presupposes a law of nature. A common basis for objection to the application of medical technology is the belief that allowing something to happen, even though we can control it technically, is to leave it to God's province, acknowledging that some circumstances are beyond our power. When suffering is reduced in smallpox, it is not usually thought of as a violation of the law of nature or divine design. Why, then, do we object to abortions which aim to prevent disability and suffering caused by severe genetic disorders? Jainas do not accept the existence of God as the creator or controller of the universe. Therefore, the objection to 'playing God' cannot be raised from their perspective, and so in Jaina philosophy, some kind of genetic engineering would not be objected to. One needs to work out the details of every case so as not to violate the basic principles of Jainism, like *ahimsa* and the doctrine of *karma*. If the termination of human life is motivated by compassion, then abortion should not be objected to either. The main aim of the whole institution of modern medical practice is to alleviate suffering, and if it is suggested that suffering needs to be removed from the society as it is considered a kind of *himsa*, then Jainism as a religion must permit abortion on compassionate grounds.

Molecular biologists have developed a variety of techniques of genetic engineering to manipulate and control the development, structure and hereditary characteristics of organisms, and it has become a serious issue when it comes to the question of modifying the human genome. But the potential benefits of genetic engineering cannot be dismissed. In the case of human genetic modification, negative engineering is generally thought to be ethically unproblematic, while positive engineering in general is not. A basic aim of therapeutic medicine is to eliminate serious disability, and genetic technologies should be welcomed by Jains. As Jainas themselves have worked out in detail, the systems of medicines and surgery are accepted as good, when put to therapeutic use. Even fasting as a mode of meditation plays a very important role in the Jaina medical system. But the situation in the bio-medical domain is not so straightforward, and the benefits and risks need to be measured constantly. On the one hand, there is no precise, universal, objective criterion that would determine what constitutes either a 'dysfunction' or an 'enhancement'. In therapeutic somatic treatment, individuals must be allowed to make informed, autonomous choices. But in the case of germ-line modifications, deciding the destiny of others without their consent is quite problematic from a moral point of view. Improving the shelf-life of tomatoes does not generate much of a problem, but tinkering with the complex system of the human genome may involve serious problems. So in which areas should genetic engineering be allowed, and where should one stop? This is a question to which there is no ready answer. Organ transplantation would in general not be accepted in the Jaina system of thought, as it is considered *himsa*. Prolonging the 'natural life' of human beings is an ideal, but by having less and less, by maintaining austerity and self-discipline. Cloning, changing one's sex, etc., are not welcomed by Jainas, as this is interfering with the *karma* principle. One cannot change the *karmic* flow of any being; the moral status of all living beings is equal, and they all lie within the scope of morality.

With regard to the notion of justice and fair distribution of resources for health care, the Jaina perspective always treats this as an ideal, and an organisational need that is much welcomed. At the individual level, though, one must not possess more than what is necessary for one's basic needs (*aparigraha*), and 'fair distribution' is decided by individuals themselves (through the moral codes for the layman).

The most important thing in this context is: the interest of the individual concerned and the interest of the 'others'; the right of the concerned individual to die or to live; and the responsibility or moral obligation of 'others' towards living beings or the human embryo, foetus, and the newborn. Jainism advocates that all living beings have equal autonomy, freedom, and a right to live, and in some circumstances, a right to die (as we have discussed with reference to *sallekhana*). With regard to euthanasia, *sallekhana* is accepted; socially, it is not considered suicide, but allowing the body to die gradually with the help of a monk when the body becomes a hindrance in attaining liberation. It is a very long and carefully worked-out process, which has to be followed strictly. It is one thing to allow someone to die after living a full life, and something else to remove the life-support system due to certain constraints, financial or otherwise. Here, too, one has to carefully work out the complexities of the situation and come to a conclusion. 'Killing' is *himsa* and not allowed at any cost, but 'letting someone die' in some circumstances is permitted within the Jaina framework, both in the individual and social interest.

To conclude, I have tried to respond to some of the bio-ethical issues following Jaina philosophy, its logic, principles and method. Jainas use a dialectical method, which is carefully worked out between 'God' and universe, *ekanta* and *anekanta,* monk and layman, spiritual and practical, a monk's obligation and a layman's obligation, individual obligation and social obligation, and freedom and determination. This is just an attempt to begin an Indic response to the bio-ethical issues we face the world over.

Notes

1. Some Jaina thinkers like Hemachandra (*Pramanamimamsa*) think that *anekantavada* and *syadvada* are the same thing; however, we have textual evidence in support of our interpretation. There are 24 synonyms of *anekantavada* and no two are the same, such as *akulvada* (not focused), *sankirnavada* (converging in one), *sanghatvada* (collection like grapes), *sakalvada*, etc. (Suri 1986).
2. The Jaina texts, though, do not make it clear why only these seven, and why they cannot be reduced to a smaller number of alternatives (see Bhargava 1968).
3. *Syadvada* neither leads to, nor can be equated with, *samsayavada*, as critics believe. Kundakunda says that all of us have a two-fold consciousness — *jnanacetana* (knowledge consciousness) and *karmacetana* (action consciousness) (Bhargava 1968: 33).

References

Amritachandra. 1953. *Purusarthasiddhyupaya*. Mumbai, Paramásruta prabhāvaka Mandala.

Bhargava, D. 1968. *Jaina Ethics.* Delhi: Motilal Banarasidass.

———. 1973. *The Jaina Tarka Bhasha of Acharya Yashovijaya*. Delhi: Motilal Banarasidass.

Devanandi, Pujapada. 1955. *Sarvartha-siddhi*, Pt. Phoolachandra Siddhantashastri (ed.). Varanasi: Bharatiya Jnanapitha.

Jaina Sutras Translated from the Prakrit: Part I: The Acaranga Sutra. 1989. Herman Jacobi (trans.). Delhi: Motilal Banarasidass.

Jaini, P. S. 2000. *Collected Papers on Jaina Studies*. New Delhi: Motilal Banarasidass.

Lalvani, K. C. 1973. *Dasavaikalika Sutra of Arya Sayyambhava*. Delhi: Motilal Banarasidass.

Matilal, B. K. 1981. *The Central Philosophy of Jainism (Anekānta-vāda)*. Ahmedabad: L. D. Institute of Indology.

Potter, V. R. 1975. 'Humility with Responsibility — A Bioethics for Oncologists: Presidential Address', *Cancer Research*, 35: 2297–306.

Suri, Haribhadra. 1986. *Sad-Darsana-Samuccaya*, K. Satchidanada Murty (trans.). New Delhi: Eastern Book Linkers.

Umasvati. 2002. *Tattvartha Sutra: That Which Is*, Nathmal Tatia (trans.). New Delhi: Institute of Jainology/HarperCollins.

Eleven

'Yogi-doctors' and Occult Healing Arts

Holistic Therapeutics at Sri Aurobindo Ashram

Makarand R. Paranjape

In this chapter, I attempt a post-colonial reading of healing that documents a significant therapeutic practice reported from the Sri Aurobindo Ashram.[1] The period under analysis covers the formative years of the Ashram, from the 1930s to the 1960s, when it was presided over by its masters, first Sri Aurobindo and the Mother together, and then, after the death of the former in 1950, by the latter. The Sri Aurobindo Ashram was a community that grew around the charismatic yogi, poet, philosopher, and former political revolutionary, Sri Aurobindo (1872–1950). After his studies in England from 1879–1893, Sri Aurobindo returned to India to work with Sayaji Rao Gaekwar, the ruler of Baroda, a princely state in British India. In 1906 he joined active politics following the partition of Bengal, quitting his position with the Baroda state. After a stormy and eventful, though brief, political career, some of which was spent in the Alipur jail, he quit politics in 1910, arriving on 4 April to Pondicherry (now Puducherry), then a French enclave near Madras (now Chennai) in south India.

Following several years of intense yogic practices and prolific writing, a spiritual community was formalised around him in 1920, triggered by the final arrival on 24 April 1920 of the Mother (Mirra Alfassa, 1878–1973), his spiritual partner. The Mother was born in Paris to Turkish-Egyptian Jewish parents. She was an immensely gifted and precocious spiritualist, occultist, artist, and administrator. By the time she arrived in Pondicherry, she was also widely travelled, having lived in Algeria and later in Japan. In 1968, the Mother went on to found Auroville, a city for humanity, made up of people from many nationalities and cultures.[2]

This account may be regarded as a contribution to a kind of 'salvage ethnography',[3] but with a difference. The culture and worldview that

I seek to document does not belong to endangered indigenous peoples, but to a modern, even futuristic, spiritual cult. Yet, the 'knowledge' on health and healing embodied in the practice of this movement not only bears a close resemblance to submerged and occult traditions in both the East and the West, but also to the main indigenous system of health care in India, namely Ayurveda. The latter, along with many other indigenous systems of healing, has had to both adapt and transform itself in the face of the dominance of modern bio-medicine in order to survive. In the latter portion of my argument, I turn to the relationship between Sri Aurobindo and Mother's theories of healing, and both Ayurveda and modern bio-medicine.

In addition, I consider this chapter 'post-colonial' in at least two senses. First, in its concern with the textuality of healing practices, my account is really an interpretation of a rich archive of narratives. It is, in other words, about 'stories' of healing and how we read them, not just about the substance of the stories. Second, not only am I concerned with the 'narrativity' of these healing practices, but I also read them in terms of their power relations to dominant bio-medical therapeutics and the now subaltern indigenous systems. I regard such a toggling of power and textuality as typically post-colonial. The 'post' is not just post-colonialism or post-modernism, but in other 'post-al' perspectives hinges on the 'linguistic turn'. Here, too, my attempt focuses on the discursivity of these healing practices. Indeed, the content and its 'scientific' value are not my primary concern. I engage with them only insofar as they present alternative paradigms of knowledge or contending epistemologies. My reading is thus post-colonial because I see these stories as examples of 'insurgent knowledges', or what Michel Foucault called the 'insurrection of subjugated knowledges' in the first of his 'Two Lectures' (1980: 81). According to Foucault, these 'subjugated knowledges' are often 'naive knowledges, located low down on the hierarchy, beneath the required levels of cognition and scientificity' (ibid.: 82).

In this case, interestingly, these 'insurgent knowledges' were resurrected, enunciated, further developed, and propped up by the personal authority of the gurus. Eventually, they became part of a 'magico-religious system' centred on the vast output of the gurus, studied and perpetuated by the Ashram community. Thus, my own anthropology of this healing practice draws on this specific archive, trying at the same time to read it cross-culturally so as to make it available to a larger body of interested interlocutors.

An Introduction to the Therapeutic Practices at Sri Aurobindo Ashram

If we wish to get to the essence of Sri Aurobindo's and the Mother's ideas on health and healing, we could examine how, according to them, both disease and cure occur. The Mother said that disease is basically an outcome of disequilibrium in the body: 'all illness without any exception ... is the expression of a break in equilibrium' (2003: 4). Similarly, the cure is really a matter of restoring the balance that has been disturbed:

> After all, an illness is only a wrong attitude taken by some part of the body.
>
> The chief role of the doctor is, by various means, to induce the body to recover its trust in the Supreme Grace (ibid.: 103).

The Mother is clear that the role of medicines is secondary; actually, it is the body that heals itself: 'In most cases the use of medicines ... is simply to help the body to have confidence. It is the body that heals itself. When it wants to be cured, it is cured' (2003: 105). These statements were made by the Mother on 5 June 1957. Eight years later, on 20 December 1965, she reiterates them even more emphatically:

> In every case, it is the Force that cures.
>
> Medicines have little effect; it is the faith in medicines that cures.
>
> Get treated by the doctor whom you trust and take only the medicines that inspire trust in you.
>
> The body only has trust in material methods and that is why you have to give it medicines — but medicines have an effect only if the Force acts through them.
>
> Allopaths ordinarily cure one thing, only to the detriment of another.
>
> Ayurvedic doctors do not usually have this drawback. That is why I recommend them (1978, Vol. 15: 170).

If disturbance of equilibrium is the cause of disease and the restoration of equilibrium the cure, then an enumeration or typology of both these processes may be considered to constitute the bulk of Sri Aurobindo's and the Mother's theory of healing.

I should clarify that Sri Aurobindo and the Mother were not unacquainted with modern medicine. In fact, their vocabulary of both the disturbance and the re-establishment of bodily equilibrium, that is, of disease and its cure, may even be brought in tune not only with traditional Ayurvedic ideas, but also with current scientific and allopathic practice. Nevertheless, their approach to both disease and healing is radically different. To cite a telling example of this difference, for the Mother, even disease-causing microbes are manifestations of negative vital energies: 'The microbe is a very material expression of something living in a subtle physical world' (2006: 32). What at first may sound outlandish, if not occult, is part of a larger theory which is internally consistent and unapologetic. In fact, such views, as I shall show, were not ad hoc or arbitrary, but developed over years of experience and efforts in healing. Sri Aurobindo and the Mother initiated and participated in many therapeutic experiments, in which they directed their 'spiritual' force through qualified and trained medical doctors. Their methodology consisted of a combination of the spiritual with the 'scientific', but in a manner that would be difficult for modern science to accept.

From such an overview of the broad principles, if we were to go into specifics, we would find ourselves floundering in a sea of words and ideas. This is because the collected works of Sri Aurobindo and the Mother constitute a vast archive, running into over 65 volumes. The Mother's views on healing occur in several places in her *Collected Works,* which run into 17 volumes, and are also scattered through the 13-volume *Agenda* which Satprem edited. Sri Aurobindo's ideas on this subject, though not as voluminous, are significant in that they may be considered as providing the basis for the Mother's own ideas, even though it is clear that he deferred to her in these matters. The Mother's observations on various topics pertaining to the human body, although related to Sri Aurobindo's views, may be considered to form a profound, far-reaching, and independent body of knowledge on their own. Thus, the Ashram's tendency to club them together, almost as a matter of dogma, need not necessarily be followed blindly.

As the archive is so enormous, we must often resort to compilations and selections, of which there are several. While such compilations serve as a quick introduction and digest, they have the disadvantage of quoting remarks out of context. We do not know when a particular statement was made and why. In addition, the absence of a chronological arrangement affords us no understanding of how some of the ideas changed or developed over time. The Gurus' words are thus frozen and reified as if for all time in a sort of imposed coherence and consistency.

For the purposes of this chapter, I have relied mostly on two such collections, *Integral Healing* (2006), compiled from the works of Sri Aurobindo and the Mother, and *Health and Healing in Yoga* (2003), which is a selection from the Mother's works.[4] What the latter excludes, however, is the extensive new material available in the *Agenda* (1979). *Health and Healing in Yoga* arranges the Mother's ideas in four parts, 'Causes of Illness', 'Cures and Illnesses', 'Foundations of Health', and 'The Cycle of Life'. This division gives us a glimpse of the foundations of the Mother's approach to healing. Towards the end of the book, we see health and healing to be part of a much larger plan or project which the masters had embarked upon. To my mind, these two compilations serve to counterbalance the chronological and the thematic, thus becoming good, although not perfect, source books on the subject.

Rather than begin with a detailed analysis of the Gurus' views on health and healing, my strategy is to offer a more matter-of-fact account of a doctor who served as the Ashram's physician. Such an account is also more accessible to most of us, who are grounded in modern biomedical practices. It also locates the Gurus' ideas in a more practical curative, even experimental, context. The account also shows how extensive and well-documented trials in healing were carried out at the Ashram over a period of time. It thus offers us a demonstration of some of the ideas which I shall return to later.

Nirodbaran's Account of Experiments in Healing

In January 1930, when Nirodbaran, a trained doctor with a medical degree from the University of Edinburgh, met the Mother for the first time, she asked him, 'Where do you intend to practice?' (Nirodbaran 1994: 1). He replied that he would settle down in his native town. The Mother seemed to approve, 'Yes, that would be good' (ibid.: 2). However, such was the force of this encounter that after spending a year and a half in medical service at Rangoon and about the same time in his native Chittagong, Nirodbaran returned to Pondicherry in 1933. He lived there for the next 73 years, dying at the age of nearly 103 years.[5]

First assigned to a variety of menial tasks, including a stint in the timber godown, he wrote to Sri Aurobindo complaining that his medical education, which had been completed at great cost, was being wasted. Sri Aurobindo replied, 'What would you say if the Mother actually proposed to you to exchange the timber-trade for medicine?' (Nirodbaran 1994: 24). He was immediately transferred to the Ashram Dispensary. As British subjects, doctors from India could not practice in Pondicherry, which was a French territory. The French government had, however, given permission to Ashramite-doctors to practice within the Ashram's premises. This is how Nirodbaran came to be not only Sri Aurobindo's scribe and personal physician, but also the keeper of the longest correspondence with Sri Aurobindo, which run into over 4,000 letters, many of which were published in *Correspondence with Sri Aurobindo* in two volumes.

The procedure followed at the Dispensary was that serious or complicated cases were to be referred to the local hospital, but all routine illnesses were handled by Nirodbaran. He would send detailed medical reports to the Mother, which were always read very carefully before instructions were issued. These latter were conveyed by Sri Aurobindo in his letters to Nirodbaran, but 'all instructions relating to practical questions about sadhana and work were given by the Mother' (Nirodbaran 1994: 24). In 1937, after Sri Aurobindo's eyesight weakened, the Mother herself took on the onus of the medical correspondence. In 1938, after Sri Aurobindo's accident, Nirodbaran was called upon to attend to him, thus ending his stint in the Dispensary and the medical correspondence. Even so, his connection with the Dispensary did not cease completely. When Sri Aurobindo's condition stabilised, Nirodbaran resumed attending to Ashram patients when he was off duty.

All told, Nirodbaran's work at the Ashram Dispensary was highly illuminating from a medical point of view. As he himself admits, '[a]bout the medical treatment I had a lot to learn. In fact, it was in the Mother's School that I took initiation in the Healing Art' (Nirodbaran 1994: 24–25). According to Nirodbaran, the Mother's 'knowledge of medicine was far beyond any average intelligent doctor's' (ibid.: 25). Although the source of this knowledge was 'primarily intuitive', it was 'also partly derived from her vast general experience' (ibid.).

Nirodbaran began, as any ordinary medical doctor would, with 'only the British Pharmacopoeia with its thousands of drugs and their curative properties' (Nirodbaran 1994: 26). Gradually, however, he learned that what his 'orthodox medical mind' (ibid.) knew was rather inadequate. He says,

> I had to forget or change many of my accustomed notions about drugs and stop or be careful about their use. I had to learn to employ as few medicines as possible and thereby give Nature a chance to heal (Nirodbaran 1994: 26).

Sri Aurobindo himself sent Nirodbaran an article by a famous medical authority who had been the President of the Royal College of Physicians, in which the latter 'advocated the theory that Nature cures 90–99% of our diseases and that medical practitioners are only agents of Nature' (ibid.). We have already seen that Sri Aurobindo and the Mother were rather conservative when it came to administering drugs and medications to patients. Similarly, 'as a rule, the Mother was not well-disposed towards operations' (ibid.: 28). In the course of time, Nirodbaran made a great discovery:

> it is not the germs that cause the disease, nor the drugs that cure it but the doctor — that is, the man, the personality — that counts. In other words, the doctor is an instrument of a higher Force that uses him, and medicines play a secondary role (ibid.: 26).

The result is that Nirodbaran tried, at some risk of criticism, to be a 'yogi-doctor': 'I withheld drugs for simple maladies and left the patients to their faith or inner resistance' (ibid.: 28). Speaking about the causes of illness, or what in medical parlance may be called the etiology of disease, Nirodbaran observes:

> I further learnt that behind illnesses also there are forces. These forces, psychological or occult, attack first of all the subtle sheath that envelops the body and weaken it. Then only germs can produce an illness. Anyone who has a strong and sound sheath can go about in germ-infested areas during epidemics and will be immune to any contagion or infection (ibid.: 26).

He admits, however, that he does not know

> what practical use can be made of the knowledge of the subtle sheath. A patient, if he is perceptive, can feel an attack coming upon him and ward it off in time before it enters his body, but what will be the doctor's role in it unless he too is an occultist and helps the patient in an occult way? (ibid.: 27).

His greatest lesson was that 'spiritual Force can cure diseases'. This does not mean that Nirodbaran totally suspended his scepticism or the rationality of his scientific training:

> Though I believed in it, my outer medical being probably lacked a total faith. Or else my doubting nature stood in the way and I had to put up with the Master constantly drilling my brain and pouring in more and more faith (Nirodbaran 1994: 27).

This tussle between science and spirituality, I am convinced, made Nirodbaran all the more effective as a medical practitioner.

The Mother on Disease: Its Causes and Cures

Having already introduced the Mother's basic views on disease and healing earlier, in this section I shall focus on one remarkable document, a long and involved statement delivered by the Mother on 22 July 1953, and published in the Question and Answers series of 1953 in her *Collected Works* (1978, Vol. 5: 173–81). The Mother had, on an earlier occasion (15 July 1953), assured her listeners

> [n]ext time we shall speak of health and illness and I shall confound all those who are attached by iron chains to their illness who do not want to let it go! I shall give them scissors to cut their chains (ibid.: 166).

This was that promised deliverance. It is a fairly long statement, which starts with general observations and principles, then moves to specific topics and instances, and is very rich in narrative content because it contains a detailed story of the Mother's experience of surviving an epidemic in Japan.

To begin, the Mother says quite unequivocally that 'all illness without any exception — without exception — is the expression of a break in equilibrium' (ibid.: 173):

> (I would add even accidents) come from a break in equilibrium. That is, if all your organs, all the members and parts of your body are in harmony with one another, you are in perfect health. But if there is the slightest imbalance anywhere, immediately you get either just a little ill or quite ill, even very badly ill, or else an accident occurs. That always happens whenever there is an inner imbalance (ibid.).

Then she goes on to differentiate the kinds of break in equilibrium, which she divides into the physical, vital and mental:

> But then, to the equilibrium of the body, you must add the equilibrium of the vital and the mind. For you to be able to do all kinds of things with immunity, without any accident happening to you, you must have a triple equilibrium — mental, vital, physical — and not only in each of the parts, but also in the three parts in their mutual relations. If you have done a little mathematics, you should have been taught how many combinations that makes and what a difficult thing it means! There lies the key to the problem. For the combinations are innumerable, and consequently the causes of illness too are innumerable, the causes of accidents also are innumerable. Still, we are going to try to classify them so that we may understand (1978, Vol. 5: 173).

We can see how the Mother starts with relatively simple principles, but builds them into a system capable of addressing the complexities of the actual reality.

When it comes to the physical loss of equilibrium, the Mother posits two categories: 'First of all, from the point of view of the body — just the body — there are two kinds of disequilibrium: functional and organic' (ibid.: 173). The first results from an individual organ being in disequilibrium, and hence, diseased. But even if all the organs are in themselves in good condition, the lack of proper balance between them would result in a 'functional imbalance', which can also make a person ill (ibid.: 174). According to the Mother, functional imbalances are easier to cure, while an afflicted organ is harder to treat or set right. Much of CAM therapeutics is addressed to the functional imbalance. It would seem that organic diseases respond better to allopathy, although even in this type of cure it helps to address functional issues.

Further, the Mother divides the causes of the imbalance into two, internal and external (ibid.: 174). An internal imbalance can occur if one of the organs starts malfunctioning:

> Suppose for example, your heart begins to throb madly; then you must make it calm, you tell it that this is not the way to behave, and at the same time (solely to help it) you take in long, very regular rhythmic breaths, that is, the lung becomes the mentor of the heart and teaches it how to work properly (ibid.: 175).

In this case, balance is restored through a conscious effort directed at the lungs or the breathing apparatus, which in turn tutors the heart to beat more slowly. This is the most frequent sort of inner disturbance that can cause illness. But the Mother also identifies another, the resistance of one part of the body while the others are willing to progress in Yoga:

> There is an aspiration within you (I am now speaking of people who do yoga or at any rate know what the spiritual life is and try to walk on the path), within you there is a part of the being — either mental or vital or sometimes even physical — that has understood well, has much aspiration, its special aptitudes, that receives the forces well and is making good progress. And then there are others that cannot, others still that don't want to (that of course is very bad), but there are yet others that want to very much but cannot, do not have the capacity, are not ready. So there is something that rises upward and something that does not move. That causes a terrible imbalance. And usually this translates itself into some illness or other, for you are in such a state of inner tension between something that cannot or something that clings, that does not want to move and something else that wants to: that produces a frightful unease and the result usually is an illness (1978, Vol. 5: 175–76).

There is also the case of the whole being advancing, except for a small part which is resistant:

> Now there is the opposite, almost the opposite, that is, the whole being goes ahead, progresses, advances in an increasing equilibrium and achieves remarkable progress; you have the feeling you are in a wonderfully favourable state, everything is going on well, you are sure; and you see yourself already gloriously well on the way. Crack! An illness. Then you say: 'How is it? I was in such a good condition and now I have fallen ill! It is not fair.' But this happens because you are not completely conscious. There was a small part in the being that did not want to move. Usually it is something in the vital; sometimes it is a tiny mental formation that does not agree to follow; sometimes it is simply something in the body which is quite inert or has not the slightest intention of moving, that wants things to remain always as they are. It pulls backward, separates itself wilfully, and naturally, even if it is quite small, it brings about such an imbalance in the being that you fall ill (ibid.: 176).

Or:

> somewhere in your being — either in your body or even in your vital or mind, either in several parts or even in a single one — there is an incapacity to receive the descending Force, this acts like a grain of sand in a machine. You know, a fine machine working quite well with everything going all right, and you put into it just a little sand (nothing much, only a grain of sand), suddenly everything is damaged and the machine stops . . . There was something that could not receive; immediately it brings about a disequilibrium. Even though very small it is enough, and you fall ill (Mother 1978, Vol. 5: 178).

Overall, the Mother holds that illnesses often have causes other than purely physical ones:

> the illness had another cause than the purely physical one; there was another. The first was only an outer expression of a different disorder, and unless you touched that, discovered that disorder, never would you be able to prevent the illness from coming (ibid.: 179).

Such is an overview of the internal causes of disturbance.

Coming to the external causes, the Mother says that sometimes, though one may be internally in perfect balance, the external surroundings may be 'full of imbalance' (ibid):

> [Y]ou are obliged to receive what comes from outside. You give and you receive; you breathe in and absorb . . . [F]or you live in a state of ceaseless vibrations. You give out your vibrations and receive also the vibrations of others, and these vibrations are of a very complex kind . . . You give, you receive; you give, you receive. It is a perpetual play . . . all is contagious, everything (ibid.: 179–80).

In such a situation, those who are hyper-sensitive are bound to absorb the external disturbances. So a person can become ill even if there is no active negativity in the environment, just through the disequilibrium in the world outside.

But the Mother also identifies active ill-will: 'Unhappily there is much bad will in the world' (ibid.: 180). Again, there are two types. Sometimes its carriers are themselves unconscious: 'Unintentionally . . . others are attacked, they don't know, they pass it on without even being aware of it. They are the first victims. They pass the illness to others . . .' (ibid.).

While some people are unwitting mediums of such ill-will, there are others who are wilfully wicked:

> There is a misguided, perverted occultism which is called black magic, it is a thing one must never touch. But unfortunately, there are people who touch it through pure wickedness. You must not believe it is an illusion, a superstition; it is real. There are people who know how to do magic and do it, and with their magic they obtain altogether detestable results (1978, Vol. 5: 180).

That is why the Mother insists that a sincere practitioner of yoga must never harbour negative thoughts about others: 'All who do yoga sincerely must . . . never . . . have bad will or a bad thought towards others' (ibid.: 181).

It is now that the Mother comes up with her explanation of how microbes are created:

> [T]here are in the physical atmosphere, the earth-atmosphere, numerous small entities which you do not see . . . Some of them are quite nice, others very wicked. Generally these little entities are produced by the disintegration of vital beings — they pullulate — and these form quite an unpleasant mass . . . They like little accidents, they like the whole whirl of forces that gather round an accident: a mass of people . . . And then that gives them their food, because, in reality, they feed upon human vitality thrown out of the body by emotions and excitements (ibid.: 181–82).

The worst of these are 'forces of disintegration' which, according to the Mother, 'is the origin of germs and microbes' (ibid.: 181):

> [M]ost microbes have behind them a bad will and that is what makes them so dangerous. And unless one knows the quality and kind of bad will and is capable of acting upon it, there is a ninety-nine per cent chance of not finding the true and complete remedy. The microbe is a very material expression of something living in a subtle physical world . . . . The origin of the microbes and their support lie in a disharmony, in the being's receptivity to the adverse force (ibid.).

After this explanation of the origin of microbes, the Mother proceeds to narrate an extraordinary story of her own encounter with an epidemic in Japan at the beginning of January 1919:[6]

> it was the time when a terrible flu raged there in the whole of Japan, which killed hundreds of thousands of people. It was one of those

> epidemics the like of which is rarely seen. In Tokyo, every day there were hundreds and hundreds of new cases. The disease appeared to take this turn: it lasted three days and on the third day the patient died. And people died in such large numbers that they could not even be cremated . . . if one did not die on the third day, at the end of seven days one was altogether cured . . . There was a panic in the town, for epidemics are very rare in Japan. They are a very clean people, very careful and with a fine morale. Illnesses are very rare. But still this came, it came as a catastrophe (Mother 1978, Vol. 5: 181–82).

The Mother often wonders, 'What is there behind this disease?' (ibid.). For a while she is fine, but one day she is called to the other end of town. When she returns, she has caught it:

> I had to cross the whole town in a tram-car. And I was in the tram and seeing these people with masks on their noses, and then there was in the atmosphere this constant fear . . . I came to the house, I passed an hour there and I returned. And I returned with a terrible fever. I had caught it. It came to you thus, without preparation, instantaneously (ibid.: 183).

The doctor is called, but the Mother refuses his medicine. She remains in bed, thinking 'What is this illness? Why is it there? What is there behind it?' (ibid.: 184). Then she finds out:

> At the end of the second day, as I was lying all alone, I saw clearly a being, with a part of the head cut off, in a military uniform (or the remains of a military uniform) approaching me and suddenly flinging himself upon my chest, with that half a head to suck my force. I took a good look, then realised that I was about to die. He was drawing all my life out (for I must tell you that people were dying of pneumonia in three days). I was completely nailed to the bed, without movement, in a deep trance. I could no longer stir and he was pulling. I thought: now it is the end. Then I called on my occult power, I gave a big fight and I succeeded in turning him back so that he could not stay there any longer. And I woke up (ibid.).

The Mother now relates this to her earlier experiences:

> But I had seen. And I had learnt, I had understood that the illness originated from beings who had been thrown out of their bodies. I had seen this during the First Great War, towards its end, when people used to live in trenches and were killed by bombardment. They were

> in perfect health, altogether healthy and in a second they were thrown out of their bodies, not conscious that they were dead. They did not know they hadn't a body any more and they tried to find in others the life they could not find in themselves. That is, they were turned into so many countless vampires. And they vampirised upon men. And then over and above that, there was a decomposition of the vital forces of people who fell ill and died. One lived in a kind of sticky and thick cloud made up of all that. And so those who took in this cloud fell ill and usually got cured, but those who were attacked by a being of that kind invariably died, they could not resist (Mother 1978, Vol. 5: 184–85).

Although this being was 'irresistible', the Mother had the occult knowledge and power to overcome it. After a few days, the Mother is told by a visitor that the epidemic has abated. When the Mother narrates her story to her friend, he goes and tells it to many others, so much so that '[t]hey even published articles about it in the papers' (ibid.: 185). Unfortunately, these newspaper reports have not yet been found.

This extraordinary account resembles a mythological narrative such as the Devi Mahatmyaham or the 'Glory of the Goddess', a popular religious text extolling the victory of the Devi over Mashisasura or the 'Buffalo demon'. Also called the 'Chandi Path' or simply Chandi, this narrative of 700 verses extracted from the longer Markandeya Purana (c. 500 CE) is read ritualistically by devotees as a way of worshipping the Goddess. At its heart, it is a triumphant account of the feminine deity disciplining, overcoming, and finally beheading the hypermasculine fiend (see Coburn 1991). The text recounts heroic battles between the Goddess and her demonic adversaries; each story illustrates a different aspect of the Devi's divinity — Mahakali in Chapter 1, Mahalakshmi in Chapters 2–4, and Mahasaraswati in Chapters 5–13. It is these precise names of the Goddess that Sri Aurobindo himself invokes in his celebrated text, 'The Mother', adding to it Maheshwari, another emanation or aspect of the Goddess. Originally written in the form of letters in 1927, a revised version of this text is standard reading for the followers of Sri Aurobindo and the Mother. Not only does the book describe the Divine Goddess, but later Sri Aurobindo also explicitly identified the head of the Ashram, the Mother, with the former.[7] It is thus a text that deifies the Mother, making her a living Goddess. In narrating her account of her victory over the Influenza Demon, the

Mother is thus performing her Goddess function in the same tradition as texts like the Chandi.

Having enumerated both the internal and the external causes of illness, the Mother now comes to the cure. The body must be convinced that 'it has been given the conditions under which it must be all right', so that 'it takes the resolution that it must be all right and it is cured' (Mother 1978, Vol. 5: 186). According to her, there are people 'ill out of spite, there are people who are ill out of hate, there are people who are ill through despair' (ibid.), so what is most important is to have a very high degree of self-awareness and scrutiny to find out which part of one's body is actually open to or harbours illness. Once the disharmony has been discovered, 'the first thing to do is to quieten oneself, bring peace, calm, relaxation, with a total confidence, in this little corner (not necessarily in the whole body)':

> Afterwards you see what is the cause of the disorder. You look. Of course, there are many, but still you try to find out approximately the cause of this disorder, and through the pressure of light and knowledge and spiritual force you re-establish the harmony (ibid.).

In more difficult or stubborn cases, the Mother says:

> you must add the Force of spiritual purification which is such an absolutely perfectly constructive force that nothing that's in the least destructive can survive there. If you have this Force at your disposal or if you can ask for it and get it, you direct it on the spot and the adverse force usually runs away immediately, for if it happens to be in the midst of this Force it gets dissolved, it disappears; for no force of disintegration can survive within this Force; therefore disintegration disappears and with it that also disappears. It can be changed into a constructive force, that is possible, or it may be simply dissolved and reduced to nothing. And with that not only is the illness cured, but all possibility of its return is also eliminated. You are cured of the illness once and for all, it never comes back (ibid.: 187–88).

Finally, the Mother implies that prevention is better than cure. To prevent disease, one must not allow it to affect one's physical body. In an earlier session on 16 June 1929, the Mother had explained that

> To whatever cause an illness may be due, material or mental, external or internal, it must, before it can affect the physical body, touch another

> layer of the being that surrounds and protects it. This subtler layer is called in different teachings by various names — the etheric body, the nervous envelope . . . All communications with the exterior world are made through this medium, and it is this that must be invaded and penetrated first before the body can be affected. If this envelope is absolutely strong and intact, you can go into places infested with the worst of diseases, even plague and cholera, and remain quite immune. It is a perfect protection against all possible attacks of illness (Mother 1978, Vol. 3: 89).

But what is this 'etheric body' or 'nervous envelope'? It is

> built up, on the one side, of a material basis, but rather of material conditions than of physical matter, on the other, of the vibrations of our psychological states. Peace and equanimity and confidence, faith in health, undisturbed repose and cheerfulness and bright gladness constitute this element in it and give it strength and substance. It is a very sensitive medium with facile and quick reactions; it readily takes in all kinds of suggestions and these can rapidly change and almost remould its condition. A bad suggestion acts very strongly upon it; a good suggestion operates in the contrary sense with the same force. Depression and discouragement have a very adverse effect; they cut out holes in it, as it were, in its very stuff, render it weak and unresisting and open to hostile attacks an easy passage (Mother 1978, Vol. 3: 89).

Speaking more than 30 years later, on 27 January 1951, the Mother repeats her theory:

> The vital body surrounds the physical body with a kind of envelope . . . It is this which protects the body from all contagion, fatigue, exhaustion and even from accidents. Therefore if this envelope is wholly intact, it protects you from everything, but a little too strong an emotion, a little fatigue, some dissatisfaction or any shock whatsoever is sufficient to scratch it as it were and the slightest scratch allows any kind of intrusion. Medical science also now recognises that if you are in perfect vital equilibrium, you do not catch illness or in any case you have a kind of immunity from contagion. If you have this equilibrium, this inner harmony which keeps the envelope intact, it protects you from everything. There are people who lead quite an ordinary life, who know how to sleep as one should, eat as one should, and their nervous envelope is so intact that they pass through all dangers as though unconcerned. It is a capacity one can cultivate in oneself. If one becomes aware of

> the weak spot in one's envelope, a few minutes' concentration, a call to the force, an inner peace is sufficient for it to be all right, get cured, and for the untoward thing to vanish (Mother 1978, Vol. 4: 59).

To conclude this section, we may go to the Mother's message on 2 July 1963 on the occasion of the inauguration of the Children's Dispensary in the Ashram:

> As many cases
> so many cures.
> The most important thing in therapeutics is to teach the body to react properly and reject the illness (Mother 1978, Vol. 15: 171).

We might consider this a superbly pithy summing up of her whole theory.

To those familiar with the philosophy of Sri Aurobindo and the Mother, this approach to healing is based on a certain understanding of the human being as consisting of five levels of being: physical, vital, mental, psychic, and spiritual. Both health and disease are thus related to all these levels. Each of these levels, in turn, has all the other elements within it, thus making for a complex and multi-tiered ladder of consciousness. When it comes to healing, the Mother explains it as follows: 'Each spot of the body is symbolical of an inner movement; there is there a world of subtle correspondences' (Mother 1978, Vol. 3: 88). Such a notion has much in common with the ancient systems of the Cabala, neo-Platonism, alchemy, and hermeticism, among others, which in turn share a certain philosophical orientation not only with Ayurveda, but also with Tibetan and Chinese medicine.

Disease, as we commonly understand it, is a physical phenomenon. Therefore, my observations in most part are confined to the first two of the five levels. Yet, it should be remembered that health and healing are only a small part of the Integral Yoga of Sri Aurobindo and the Mother, whose aim is nothing short of the total transformation of the human being and of life on earth. In the last instance, even the conquest of death is a part of the agenda. First, human consciousness must be changed radically; then the body itself altered so that it becomes a fit vehicle. This process, called supramentalisation, entails 'the end of disease, suffering (of all kinds, including material suffering) and death' (Pandey 2006: 279). Such ideas as physical transformation or the quest for immortality, although dismissed as myths by the modern mind, are prevalent in most traditions known to us. Indeed, as Richard S. Weiss's recent book *Recipes for Immortality* shows, this quest continues to inform both the worldview and practices of Siddha medicine in Tamil Nadu to this day. Modern medicine, too, is making rapid strides in not only the prolongation of life, but also in genetic modifications, which might eventually slow down the process of ageing and possibly even overcome death. It would seem, then, that such diverse paths as alchemy, occultism, spirituality, and modern science are all interested alike in this problem.

In Indian mythology, there were basically two approaches in this quest, the *asuric* and the *yogic* (Pandey 2006: 263). In the first, there was an attempt, through severe askesis and austerities, to attain physical immortality without transforming the consciousness. The attempt was to enjoy unlimited power and pleasure. These attempts were often thwarted by the Gods, with the practitioner terminated after he had exceeded a certain boundary. On the other side, the yogis too tried to increase human freedom by seeking both physical and spiritual perfection. Sri Aurobindo and the Mother's endeavour belong to the latter tradition. Modern science, with its body-centric and materialistic outlook, on the other hand, is closer to the *asuric* or demonic approach, in that it is not concerned with ethics or alteration of the consciousness. Indeed, if we turn to some works of science fiction for ways in which the future enhancement of the human potential is imagined, then we are confronted with a host of monsters — cyborgs, terminators, robots, and all kinds of strange combinations of man and machine, usually waging endless war against the precarious remnants of the human race.

According to Sri Aurobindo and the Mother, death was a spiritual necessity at a certain stage in evolution. Without it, 'imperfect forms would multiply ad infinitum as viruses and bacteria do' (Pandey 2006: 279). But when the consciousness of a species has been perfected, it will have no need to die. It would be a threat neither to itself nor to other species. Such a being would, in theory, have the 'freedom to change the body consciously by an act of will without going through the process of death' (ibid.: 280). The Mother has spoken extensively on what such a transformed and supramentalised body might be like. According to her, in traditions older than the Vedic and the Chaldean, there is

> already a mention of a 'glorious body' which would be plastic enough to be transformed at every moment by the deeper consciousness: it would

> express that consciousness, it would have no fixity of form (quoted in Pandey 2006: 280).

The Mother wonders if there ever were such beings on earth, but asserts that 'in a very small way there have been partial instances of one thing or another, examples which go to prove that it is possible' (quoted in ibid.: 281). Based on these, she says that 'one could go so far as to conceive of the replacement of material organs and their functioning as it now is, by centres of concentration of force and energy which would be receptive to the higher forces' (ibid.). She goes on to offer a preliminary description of what a supramentalised body might be like:

> The supramental body which has to be brought into being here has four main attributes: lightness, adaptability, plasticity and luminosity. When the physical body is thoroughly divinised, it will feel as it were always walking on air, there will be no heaviness or *tamas* or unconsciousness in it. There will also be no end to its power of adaptability: in whatever conditions it is placed it will immediately be equal to the demands made upon it because its full consciousness will drive out all that inertia and incapacity which usually make Matter a drag to the Spirit. Supramental plasticity will enable it to stand the attack of every hostile force which strives to pierce it . . . Lastly, it will be turned into the stuff of light, each cell will radiate the supramental glory. Not only those who are developed enough to have their subtle sight open but the ordinary man too will be able to perceive this luminosity. It will be an evident fact to each and all, a permanent proof of the transformation which will convince even the most sceptical (quoted in ibid.: 282–83).

I have brought in these dimensions at the end because they are somewhat outside the scope of its main thrust, that is, traditional systems of medicine and healing. However, we must remember that these systems are a total package in which healing is only a small part. To access only the latter is, perhaps, to do violence to the system. On the other hand, as modern people, we cannot go the whole hog with some of these systems, because they stretch our capacity to suspend disbelief. Sometimes, it is hard to tell when something is plausible and when it tips over into the realm of the incredible and the fantastic.

Ashram Therapeutics and Ayurveda

Before closing, I would like to contextualise this narrative from the Sri Aurobindo Ashram, locating it in broader traditions of complimentary and alternate medicine. Such a move not only makes this account seem less outlandish or implausible, but is also not altogether at variance with the premises of age-old healing systems, which have still not been banished from our midst or relegated to the dustbin of history. Indeed, considerable attention and importance has been paid in even the discipline of medical anthropology to what were termed 'magico-religious' systems of health care. For instance, working on Japan, Margaret Lock (1980) makes a distinction between 'East Asian medicine', based on traditional Chinese medicine, and modern 'cosmopolitan medicine', or contemporary Western-style bio-medicine. In addition, there is 'folk medicine', which refers to the residual Shinto practices. In Aurobindo Ashram, too, in addition to Sri Aurobindo's and the Mother's use of the occult 'spiritual Force' to heal, there are modern medical practices, in addition to homeopathy clinics, naturopaths, Ayurvedic practitioners, and so on. The Ashram community and Auroville are busy hubs of several complimentary, at times contending, healing systems. Together, they constitute a 'holistic' or integral model of health care and healing.

My particular emphasis in this section, however, is on Ayurveda, the leading healing system to modern bio-medicine as far as India is concerned. According to some studies, nearly 80 per cent of India's over 1.2 billion people still depend on Ayurveda. While many studies have focused on the dubious safety or toxicity of Ayurvedic medicines, especially those marketed through websites (see, for instance, Gogtay et al. 2006), my concern here is with its underlying philosophy of disease and healing. It is that which connects it with the Aurobindonian narratives discussed here, and with other complementary and alternative medical systems.

What, then, is Ayurveda (see Morrison 1995 for a useful introduction)? Literally, it is a combination of two Sanskrit words, *ayush*, which means life, health, or well-being, and *veda*, which means knowledge, science, or guide. Together, the words may be taken to mean a total system for ensuring good health and a long life; David Frawley, in *Ayurvedic Healing*, calls it 'the science of life' (2003: 6). Ayurveda is India's traditional medical system. It is perhaps the most extensive, continuous, and well-known system, but is certainly not the only one. In the south, especially in Tamil Nadu, another system called Siddha is well-established, going back, like Ayurveda, to mythical times. There are also other systems in use, for example the Unani or the traditional Islamic medicine in India. Unani means Greek; so presumably this was a Arabic adaptation and development of the Greek system that also gave rise to modern medicine in the West. In addition, India has practitioners of Tibetan medicine, which shows influences of both Ayurveda and Chinese medicine, and of Homeopathy, a comparatively recent import from the West. There are, moreover, many other kinds of non-standard, non-systematised healing systems such as Indian versions of shamanism and exorcism, not to mention several forms of New Age healing, and so on. All these systems coexist with modern medicine, which though dominant, has not been able to displace or destroy the other systems altogether.

One of my concerns has been how to mediate between these systems and practices and modern or 'scientific' medicine. Certainly, in its stress on balance, prevention, and mind–body–spirit holism, the Aurobindo Ashram experiments in healing bear family resemblances with some of the alter-scientific traditional systems mentioned above. I say 'alter-scientific' because I am excluding approaches to healing which are either non-systematic, or lacking in sufficient scientific data. Some examples of the latter are aromatherapy, gemology, reiki, pranic healing, shamanism, and so on. My focus has been on how the Ashram experiment related to the traditional systems with long histories of theory and practice on the one hand, and with modern bio-medicine on the other.

In dealing with this question, I was confronted with a curious paradox. On the one hand we can find that in the West, especially in the US, there is a greater openness to 'CAM'; on the other hand, in India, even the so-called CAM practitioners often prescribe allopathic medications. The prosperous elites in India reflect the alternative-seeking behaviour characteristic of developed countries. But the situation with the vast majority of ordinary healthcare seekers is quite different. Here, we witness a despiritualisation of healing traditions, with vast numbers of the rural population being drawn to modern medical care; even practitioners of traditional medical systems are often found prescribing allopathic medicines. Thus, the Indian situation represents the emergence of reductionism within the holistic framework of traditional medicine, while the global situation shows the emergence of holism within the reductionist framework of modern medicine.

Clearly, the Ashram experiment explicitly focused on a form of 'spiritual healing', that is, giving prominence to trans-physical aspects of the healing process. Similarly, all traditional systems of healing do not disaggregate the trans-physical from the physical. That is to say, both disease and healing have to do with more than just our bodies. Of course, here we encounter another difficulty. What do we actually mean by the word 'body'? Modern medicine, no doubt, starts with the physical, but does not rule out the other dimensions of bodily existence, including the hormonal and neurological levels, which in lay language we might call emotional or mental states. Of course, hormones and the brain are also considered purely 'physical'. They are the material mechanisms for mediating the effects of the mind. In other words, science is not closed to discovering more and more levels of the body and its consciousness, provided these fit into the picture of reality based on sensory perception. The traditional systems, on the other hand, do not start, and certainly do not end, with the body, mind or intellect. They see a person as really being a soul or a self, what in Sanskrit is called Atman. They also have a different psychology from modern medicine, actually positing not just the physical, but the subtle and the causal bodies. So what both sides mean by the 'body' is by no means the same. Both, for instance, would like to work on the 'body' — but the question is, which body and where does it end? It would appear that for modern science, all trans-physical entities and processes, including the mind and consciousness, are reducible to the body. Traditional healing practices, however, have much more complex metaphysical and ontological structures. To some, the non-corporeal entity, call it soul, psyche, or self, is more enduring than the body, even if not entirely independent of it. To others, the body actually appears in and to the self; that is, the self is primary and antecedent to the body.[8]

If we consider Ayurveda an example of the latter, we find that its entire outlook to well-being and disease is based on the notion of three biological humours, or *doshas* — *vata* (air), *pitta* (fire) and *kapha* (water). When these are out of harmony, we experience disease. The unique insight of Ayurveda is that good health is our natural state because what we really are is the Atman, immortal and untrammelled. If so, embodiment itself is akin at worst to disease, or at best, to self-limitation. From an extreme, advaitic point of view, we are non-identical with our bodies. If we are not the body, then certainly we are not whatever happens to the body, including disease. Transcending the body in our consciousness, then, is a way of being ourselves, that is, being healthy.

Luckily, for those more bodily inclined, Ayurveda does not take such a position at all. It not only accepts embodiment, but also looks for the cause of disease in the disturbance of the natural equilibrium of the body. Ayurveda also treats the body with those substances, herbal or mineral, that are part of the same natural habitat and environment as the diseased body, thereby hoping, through depletion or augmentation, to restore the harmony of the body within itself and with the rest of its surroundings. Ayurveda, however, does not stop with the body. It does not rule out other sources of both disease and therapy. The extra-physical or even cosmic forces, it believes, do impact us. So if we can propitiate or affect them in some way, we ought to. Yet, its concern is primarily with the body.

Ayurveda, like other traditional medical systems, sees the cosmos as a unity, made up of an elaborate structure of correspondences between the inner and the outer, between the human being and the world, between the microcosm and the macrocosm. The disequilibrium of one, in the strict sense, is also implicated in the disequilibrium of the rest. It is through and because of this connection or inter-relatedness that Ayurveda does not rule out therapies that claim to work on these extraneous elements. It is to this extent that astrology, psychology or personal history come into play in the therapeutic process. While taking all these factors into account, ultimately Ayurveda's principal focus remains on the body.

The theory of humours or bodily types, in some form or another, also seems common to all traditional systems, regardless of geographical location. Similarly, the idea that disease is literally that — a lack of ease — caused by disturbance or disequilibrium inside the body, appears to run through all traditional systems. The subtraction from or addition of substances to the body as a way to restore the balance, also obtains in all systems. Thus, in both the cause and cure of disease, traditional systems seem to share a common philosophical foundation.

This suggests that there was one universal system of medicine all over the world, with its local variants and techniques, just as there is one universal modern system of medicine now, with its own local variants and techniques. If we consider Jean Gebser's idea of 'structures of consciousness', then we could posit that each structure of consciousness has its own system of healing.[9] Gebser identifies four such structures, archaic, magical, mythic, and mental, which is largely our present. But he does not stop there; he goes on to aver that we are now in transition to the fifth structure, which he calls integral. In the integral structure, the other four structures need not be rejected, but can be retained or adapted for whatever they have to offer.

From such a perspective, shamanism would belong to the magic structure of consciousness, and Ayurveda and the other traditional systems, with their elaborate series of correspondences, to the mythic. After all, the humours are not meant to be taken literally, but function as archetypes. They are a tool to help us understand different constitutions and temperaments. They are a tool in diagnosis and prescription, and not some straitjacket or reductive framework. It is the modern mentality that reads them literally and thus renders them nonsensical. The non-literal and metaphorical mythical imagination does not resort to such analytical literal-mindedness or reductionism.

When we consider modern medicine, it too looks at a multiplicity of factors that might cause disease, although not in quite the same way or language as Ayurveda does:'[I]n the pathogenesis of disease, the resistance, immunity, age, and nutritional state of the person exposed, as well as virulence or toxicity of the agent and the level of exposure, all play a role' ('Human Disease' 2008: 18–19).

From an Ayurvedic point of view, all these agents and causes lead to the disequilibrium that is disease. Again, let us consider the most widely used classifications of disease in modern medicine:

> (1) topographic, by bodily region or system, (2) anatomic, by organ or tissue, (3) physiological, by function or effect, (4) pathological, by the nature of the disease process, (5) etiologic (causal), (6) juristic, by speed of advent of death, (7) epidemiological, and (8) statistical. Any single disease may fall within several of these classifications ('Human Disease' 2008: 63).

Again, it seems to me that Ayurveda would have no trouble accepting these. Indeed, an increasing number of recent studies, such as by Johannessen and Lázár (2005), are trying to understand patients and healing processes both cross-culturally and holistically, taking into account modern bio-medicine alongside alternative and traditional medical practices. What this means, at least to me, is that the two systems, the two epistemologies, the two worldviews are not entirely incompatible.

Conclusion

The integral and cross-cultural anthropology of healing that I have tried to develop here does not attempt to reconcile these differing worldviews such as the Ashram healing methods and Ayurveda on the one hand, and modern bio-medicine on the other. Rather, the effort has been to understand them as structures of consciousness, even trying to integrate them in a greater domain of human cultural understanding. Integrality does not mean sinking into irrationality or myth-making; it simply means not accepting the dominant boundaries of where valid knowledge stops and storytelling begins. That is why what I have attempted here is not a reconciliation of incommensurables, but their juxtaposition, so as to force a richer discursive terrain of sapience. One way to explain this is to make a plea for wisdom, not just reason. What this means actually is to recognise each structure for what it is — not just myth for myth and reason for reason, but also the possibility that myth may embody a form or reason, and that reason may itself work in a mythical way. Integrality recognises that we are rational, but it also knows that we are not merely or entirely rational. Therefore, it also recognises the archaic, magical, and mythic components of our being. Again, we need not take these labels literally; after all, what is not rational is not necessarily irrational or infra-rational. To be integral is to address all these, to take them into account as much as possible; and to bring to bear our knowledge of each of these in the process of healing is what the desideratum of narratives such as I have documented here seem to point towards. In the context of healing, more specifically, and of the science more generally, the science–spirituality dialogue might sometimes trigger unexpected insights. What seems both fruitful and imperative, at any rate, is the rediscovery of the ever-present integral, whose plenary possibilities may have the power and intelligence to solve our problems, and to rearrange the fragments that constitute our present limited and murky groping into lucidity or transparency.

Notes

1. The word 'Ashram' has now entered the English language. It signifies a religious retreat or spiritual community (see, for instance, Dictionary.com, 'Ashram': http://dictionary.reference.com/browse/Ashram?db=dictionary). Derived from the Sanskrit adnominal prefix *a* (near or close by) + *srama* (exertion, effort, in this case spiritual or religious). But more importantly, an Ashram is a place of spiritual instruction presided over by a Guru or teacher. In that sense, it is literally a Guru's home or establishment, where disciples gather around to learn, study, and grow spiritually.
2. For an excellent account of this unique spiritual community and its founders, see van Vrekhem (1999).

3. The term is attributed to Jacob Gruber, who used it to describe the work of 19th-century ethnographers attempting to document the languages, cultures, and worldviews of indigenous peoples on the brink of extinction or extermination by the onslaught of colonialism and modernity.
4. I must clarify that what I mean by 'integral healing' is somewhat different from what is meant by the compilers of this collection of the Mother's sayings. The latter simply call the Mother's views on healing 'integral', just as they call Sri Aurobindo's yoga 'integral'. Indeed, 'integral' is used ubiquitously for the masters' ideas on most fields, including education, psychology, sociology, and so on. If integral is a method peculiar to Sri Aurobindo and the Mother, it really means 'inclusive', that is, taking into account all the levels of being and consciousness that they identified as constituting the human being. However, by 'integral' in this chapter, I mean a way of mediating between modern medicine and alternate therapies such as Ayurveda, without rejecting or exclusively subscribing to either. How it proposes to combine, synthesise, or mediate between them is, of course, subject for another paper.
5. Born 17 November 1903; died 7:50 PM, 17 July 2006, Pondicherry.
6. The pandemic of Spanish flu or influenza referred to here began in March 1918, and lasted till June 1920. An estimated 50–100 million people died from it, making it one of the deadliest in human history. According to an article by A. Kawana and others in *Emerging Infectious Diseases*, 23 million people in Japan were infected, out of which 390,000 died.
7. See Vol. 25 of *Sri Aurobindo Birth Centenary Library*. The full text, including Sri Aurobindo's identification of the Mother with the Divine Mother, is also available at http://intyoga.online.fr/text_idx.htm (accessed 21 February 2010).
8. For an excellent cross-cultural discussion of these issues, see Ward (2004).
9. Jean Gebser's work, though still not widely known, represents a major departure from dominant modes of 20th-century Western thought. See Fuerstein (1987) and my own essay 'Nurturing Transparency: Globalization, Integrality, and Jean Gebser' (2008).

References

Aurobindo, Sri. 1972. *Sri Aurobindo Birth Centenary Library*, 30 vols. Pondicherry: Sri Aurobindo Ashram.

Coburn, Thomas B. 1991. *Encountering the Goddess: A Translation of the Devi-Mahatmya and a Study of Its Interpretation*. Albany, NY: State University of New York Press.

Foucault, Michel. 1980. 'Two Lectures', in Colin Gordon (ed.), *Power/Knowledge: Selected Interviews and Other Writings, 1972–1977*, pp. 78–108. Brighton: Harvester.

Frawley, David. 2003. *Ayurvedic Healing: A Comprehensive Guide*. New Delhi: Motilal Banarasidass.

Fuerstein, Georg. 1987. *Structures of Consciousness: The Genius of Jean Gebser: An Introduction and Critique*. Lower Lake, CA: Integral Publishing.

Gebser, Jean. 1984. *The Ever-present Origin*, Noel Barstad with Algis Mickunas (trans.). Athens, Ohio: Ohio University Press.

Gogtay, N. J., H. A. Bhatt, S.S. Dalvi, and N. A. Kshirsagar. 2002. 'The use and safety of non-allopathic Indian medicines', *Drug Safety: An International Journal of Medical Toxicology and Drug Experience*, 25 (14): 1005–19.

Gruber, Jacob. 1970. 'Ethnographic Salvage and the Shaping of Anthropology', *American Anthropologist*, New Series 72 (6): 1289–99.

'Human Disease'. 2008. *Encyclopædia Britannica Online*, http://www.britannica.com/eb/article-63220 (accessed 4 April 2013).

Johannessen, Helle and Imre Lázár (eds). 2005. *Multiple Medical Realities: Patients and Healers in Biomedical, Alternative, and Traditional Medicine*. New York: Berghahn Books.

Kawana, A., G. Naka, Y. Fujikura, Y. Kato, Y. Mizuno, T. Kondo, et al. 2007. 'Spanish influenza in Japanese Armed Forces, 1918–1920', *Emerging Infectious Diseases*, 13 (4). Available on http://www.cdc.gov/EID/content/13/4/590.htm (accessed 10 May 2010).

Lock, Margaret M. 1980. *East Asian Medicine in Urban Japan*. Berkeley: University of California Press.

Morrison, Judith H. 1995. *The Book of Ayurveda: A Holistic Approach to Health and Longevity*. New York: Simon and Schuster.

Mother, The. 1978. *The Collected Works of the Mother*, 17 vols. Pondicherry: Sri Aurobindo Ashram.

———. 1979. *Mother's Agenda,* Satprem (ed.), 13 vols. New York: Institute for Evolutionary Research.

———. 2003. *Health and Healing in Yoga*. Pondicherry: Sri Aurobindo Ashram.

———. 2006. *Integral Healing*. Pondicherry: Sri Aurobindo Ashram.

Nirodbaran. 1969. *Correspondence with Sri Aurobindo*, 2 vols. Pondicherry: Sri Aurobindo Ashram.

———. 1994. *Memorable Contacts with the Mother*. Pondicherry: Sri Aurobindo Ashram.

Pandey, Alok. 2006. *Death, Dying and Beyond*. Pondicherry: Sri Aurobindo Society.

Paranjape, Makarand R. 2008. 'Nurturing Transparency: Globalization, Integrality, and Gebser', Keynote Address for International Conference on 'Integrality: Truth, Reality and Globalisation', organised by the Jean Gebser Society in association with La Trobe University, Melbourne, Australia, 19–21 June.

van Vrekhem, Georges. 1999. *Beyond Man: The Life and Work of Sri Aurobindo and The Mother.* New Delhi: HarperCollins Publishers India.

Ward, Keith. 2004. 'The World as the Body of God: A Panentheistic Metaphor', in Philip Clayton and Arthur Peacocke (eds), *In Whom We Live and Move and Have Our Being: Panentheistic Reflections on God's Presence in a Scientific World*, pp. 62–72. Grand Rapids, MI and Cambridge, UK: William B. Eerdmans Publishing Co.

Weiss, Richard S. 2009. *Recipes for Immortality: Medicine, Religion, and Community in South India.* Oxford: Oxford University Press.

Conclusion

The Science and Spirituality of Healing[1]

Pramod Kumar: Welcome to the concluding panel discussion on the Science and Spirituality of Healing.[2] We have some very eminent panelists, whom I will introduce to you shortly.

To set the tone for today's panel discussion, I will call upon Michel Danino to give us an overview of the proceedings of the conference. Michel Danino is the Convenor for the International Forum for India's Heritage, and a guest faculty member here at Amrita and at The Indian Institute of Technology, Gandhi Nagar (IIT-G). He lectures on Indian culture, science and history. He has also authored a well-regarded book on the Indus-Sarasvati civilisation.

Michel Danino: Thank you. In this panel, you will see and hear seven of those who presented papers. There were 30 speakers altogether. But through all the presentations, certain themes came up again and again and I shall try to outline those, to my mind, of real substance. Needless to say, it is a subjective presentation.

First, I would like to point out that this exchange is a part of a series of conferences and discussions all over the world, geared towards promoting a dialogue between science and spirituality because both sides recognise that there are very valid things that the other has to offer. Therefore a dialogue, if it takes place under ideal conditions, should be fruitful and result in new perspectives.

This conference was on healing, that is, in plain English, what is normally known as 'medicine'. We want to know whether, how, and to what extent science and spirituality can meet in the field of medicine, where medicine is of course understood in the broader sense of the term, as whatever deals with health.

It is not as if such a dialogue is not already happening. There are various medical systems that have been in constant dialogue with spirituality, especially the Indian systems of medicine. If you take Ayurveda, for instance, the spiritual components of the human being are an integral part of its perspective. Ayurveda cannot dissociate the spiritual aspect from the physical aspect when a patient receives treatment. So let us say this is true of the traditional systems of medical practice. It is less true of Allopathy. Allopathy, in its theoretical framework, does not require the spiritual component of the human being, and very often does not acknowledge its existence either.

Another important difference in perspective between the Allopathic view and the traditional view is the concept of 'wholeness' in health — and this is something which was defined again and again — that traditional systems like Ayurveda, Siddha medicine, Homoeopathy (which is not exactly a traditional system of medicine, but comes very well within that ambit), and others like Acupuncture (which unfortunately was not represented in our conference, but would come within the same perspective) do not define health as simply the absence of disease, but as well-being and ultimately as being oneself. You can see that in the very definition of health we already have the germ of spirituality inhering. This is something which informed the whole conference.

Now, coming to the participants: from Allopathy, we had a number of eminent practitioners, and they came from New Delhi, from Kochi, and from other places. The beauty of the conference was that all our representatives of Allopathy acknowledged the importance of the spiritual element, agreeing that it should form part of the broad perspective of Allopathy. Some of them, like Dr Yadava, who will be one of the speakers here, emphasised that there are already feelers that Allopathy is sending patients, in India at least, to other practices. Some Allopathic hospitals are trying to integrate other practices, and it is not as if it is a closed-door system of medicine. Now, of course, this is I believe largely because we are in India, and because Allopathic practitioners in India can't help hearing about other systems, and something of, well, the Indian blood, probably resonates in them. Still, this cannot always be said of the practice of Allopathy in the West. Very often, for instance in France, a country I am still familiar with, Allopathy can be a very closed-door world, which cannot even look at the validity of other systems of medicine because it believes that it is the be-all and end-all of medicine, and anything else is just not medicine. So we have many shades in Allopathy and we have to be conscious of this. I believe we had the better shades in our conference, and that is what made the dialogue possible.

In fact, this dialogue between spirituality and science in healing became a dialogue between Allopathy as a representative of science — or rather as a discipline that claims to be a representative of science (there is a small difference) on the one hand, and on the other, that which is called CAM. That is to say, Complementary and Alternative Medicines — it is Complementary, in the sense that Allopathy magnanimously accepts that some systems can complement it. For I do not know whether an Ayurvedic physician would accept that maybe Allopathy can complement Ayurveda and may become the CAM of Ayurveda. We could speculate endlessly about these things, but at least we all agree that dialogue is essential. It is the basic starting point and it ran through all our presentations.

Now, I'll just touch upon the basic points that were made, or that were underlying many of the presentations.

One of those concerns is whether we are looking, very far in the future, at an integral system, a system that would possibly integrate all these approaches to health; it was agreed that this is not something that we can hope for immediately. It is not going to happen because there are too many deep differences in the theoretical frameworks of, say, Allopathy and Ayurveda. Even Homeopathy has a totally different theoretical framework of its own, and nobody knows today if it is at all possible to integrate all this, and if it is, then when it will happen. So, by excluding integration, which is the long-term end goal, the focus was more on cooperation, collaboration, and finding common ground. There were representatives of Ayurveda, Homoeopathy, Tibetan Medicine, Siddha Medicine, Yoga and Yogic Therapy, and even Astrology. It is possible that Astrology can be integrated in the mainstream practices of medicine, not just, say, in Ayurveda, where it is traditionally drawn upon for help, but also in Allopathy. So certain issues then came to light: how are we going to test these practices? How are we going to validate them? how are we going to subject them to conventional tests like the Randomised Controlled System that Allopathy has set for itself? Whether it always really 'tests' or 'proves' anything or not is a different issue, but how are we going to do all this? This was actually a big question, and there were deep disagreements there, because these Randomised Controlled Trials, as they are called, which are the established protocols of testing the efficacy of a medical treatment, are actually designed by Allopaths. There was a case, for instance, from Homeopathy, where someone quoted an article in *The Lancet*, one of the top medical journals in the West, where tests were conducted on Homeopathy and they all failed (Shang et al. 2005: 726–32). And therefore, the conclusion was that there is nothing to

Homeopathy and there is no point even researching further, and it is all a waste of time. The reply by the Homeopathic practitioner was, you see, our whole approach to medicine is just ignored because our approach that relies on individualisation of the diagnosis. Say, if we have 10 persons with a cold, we don't give the same medicine to all 10 persons. We will examine all the symptoms individually and we'll probably give different medicines, although they may have, apparently to an allopath, the same symptoms. So, in fact, the conclusion was that those criteria of testing dictated by Allopathy cannot be valid just like that. They will have to be totally reworked, if any validation of the other systems of medicine is to have any value.

The conclusion of all this was that, in fact, the Complementary and Alternative Systems of Medicine do not have a problem in this dialogue. They can have a dialogue, and they can also accept that Allopathy is going to work better in certain cases. It is in fact Allopathy which has a problem. This does not apply to all Allopathic practitioners; I am not making a general rule. But it is Allopathy which has difficulty grasping the world of other systems of medicine, whereas the other systems are very happy in their own frameworks and do not really have a problem. This is because Allopathy is the dominant medical system in India and the world. This is where the crux of the problem lies. This is what was repeatedly pointed out — that Allopathy is founded on a reductionist and mechanistic view of the human body and until this view is enlarged, it will have difficulty integrating the real spiritual, or let us say trans-physical, dimensions of the human being.

So we do have with us here many beautiful examples of Allopathic practitioners lecturing us on spirituality, on the need to integrate, to have compassion, for instance for the patient, to empathise with the patient, identify with the patient, and projecting — and this was very impressive, coming from Allopathic practitioners — the ideal Allopath doctor-physician as someone who has to become a yogi. But this remains a kind of individual approach; it is not the mainstream kind of Allopathy, and ideally we would all like this to become the mainstream approach. Finally, we were told that collaboration and co-operation was already happening. There are, for instance, many hospitals — Dr Yadava gave us lots of examples [of hospitals] where there are wings for Ayurveda — that believe in a collaborative approach. In Tamil Nadu, lots of government hospitals have a wing for Siddha medicine. We do not hear these things, but they are a fact. A lot of government hospitals in Tamil Nadu also have a Homeopathic wing.

So it is not as if there are always very rigid walls erected. In fact, there is a lot of cooperation already on the ground, but it is not projected in the mainstream, and there is still this dominant idea that you must first go to the allopath and only — this was also pointed out in the seminar — if you have run through 10 Allopaths and have not got relief, should you go to an Ayurvedic or Homeopathic practitioner. If the collaboration on the ground develops and grows, it can lead to a lot of satisfactory answers, and ultimately treatments, and a lot of misery could be avoided.

Now, I think one of the major conclusions — and I don't think there was anybody denying this in our seminar — was that man is a multi-dimensional being. I think this, if we must summarise in one line, was one major conclusion. Unless this conclusion is accepted, ultimately no co-operation will be fruitful, and then, of course, no integration will ever be possible. But if this is accepted, then Allopathy will automatically, let us say, be tempted to borrow the wisdom of other systems, which have, sometimes for millennia (in the case of homeopathy, just two centuries), been working on these other dimensions and which have been trying, each in its own way, to integrate them into the total system of treatment.

Any ideal medical practitioner of any branch, whether it is Ayurveda or Allopathy, should have a model of understanding how an ideal medical practitioner behaves, what he should do, how he should identify with the patient, etc. So the second major conclusion from my understanding as a layman was that in fact, a perfect doctor in any discipline has to be a yogi. He has to do a spiritual *sadhana*, or at least make the effort to not only have a constant stream of compassion and empathy for the patient, but also to enter the whole consciousness of the patient. This is a message that, to my view, could only come out of India. I do not see such a message coming out of the West. Of course, there are many valuable exercises taking place in the West, but they seem to always come to a dead end. I was telling some friends the example of acupuncture in France. Acupuncture is a very valid ancient tradition of medicine that sometimes produces stupendous results and has its own theoretical framework, which is very compatible with Ayurveda and other CAMs, but is not compatible with Allopathy. However, in France, only practitioners with Allopathic degrees are allowed to practice Acupuncture. Traditionally trained Acupuncturists are not allowed.

So we have an absurd situation where an Allopathic practitioner who does not accept the framework of Acupuncture to start with can practice it, but the one who has been trained in this traditional framework is not allowed to do so.

There you can see the walls being erected, and those walls will eventually have to be dismantled. And I think ultimately, that was what everyone was trying to say — those walls will have to go sometime. And these were the attempts to work out the meeting points between the various disciplines. This is my subjective observation of the conference.

Pramod Kumar: Thank you, Michel, for giving us a fair idea of the lines that the conference took in discussing the science and spirituality of healing. The panellists are Dr O. P. Yadava, CEO and Chief Cardiac Surgeon at the National Heart Institute (NHI) in New Delhi; *Vaidya* Dr Ram Manohar, Director of Research at the Arya Vaidya Pharmacy in Coimbatore; Dr Ramesh Bijlani from the Aurobindo Ashram, New Delhi, formerly Head of the Department at the Integral Health Clinic and of the Department of Physiology at the All India Institute of Medical Sciences (AIIMS); Dr Nisha Money, a US Air Force captain and doctor at the University of Health Sciences, Preventive Medicine and Biometrics USA, who has been introducing and teaching Yoga to the US Armed Forces; Dr Mathew Fritts, a clinical research associate of the Samueli Institute, Virginia, USA; Dr V. Sujatha, Associate Professor at the Centre for Study of Social Systems, Jawaharlal Nehru University; and lastly, Professor Makarand R. Paranjape, Professor of English at the Jawaharlal Nehru University, the main organiser of this conference. Each of the panellists is requested to express their views on select themes of the conference. First, I will request Dr O. P. Yadava to present his views on the role of traditional medicine (TM) and complementary and alternative medicine (CAM) in Allopathic medical practice.

O. P. Yadava: I will speak on the so-called possibility of the 'integration' of Allopathy and Alternative Medicine. Let me confess that I do not honestly quite understand the word integration, because it has become a fashionable term, a buzz word, a flavour of the season, something in the mould of neo-renaissance, or shall I say pseudo-renaissance. Since I do not quite understand it, I give my qualified support to this. The qualification being: if it means that the Allopathic practitioners should deliver Alternative Medicine, then my answer is a categorical 'no'. An Allopathic physician takes almost 10–12 years of post-school education to become a doctor. And if you were to learn Alternative Medicine, which also involves an equal amount of rigorous training, directly from the master or from the *guru*, then it would be impossible to integrate the two. However, if it means a meeting of the two systems under a common roof, then my answer is an equally definite 'yes'. And I say this because neither mode of treatment is the be-all and end-all of what we know. Each has its problems and deficiencies. We know that in Allopathy, we can provide fairly good medical care for the structural and mechanical disorders of the body. But we have nothing for chronic disorders, or in cases where the causation is not known or may lie in the 'sixth dimension', and for end-of-life issues; we appreciate that these conditions may be better addressed by Alternative Medicine.

It is wonderful that there is a meeting ground for both, as one system's deficiencies could become the strong point for the other, and vice-versa. Allopathy has a lot to learn from Alternative Medicine; the tenets of a good doctor–patient relationship, the concept of divine grace or preceptor's good, the concept of healing as opposed to cure, empathy against sympathy, the healing power of touch, etc. — we can certainly apply some of these in Allopathy. Now, these concepts relevant to Allopathy have been mentioned in our scriptures, but we have lost them today. In collaboration, Ayurveda can help us and we can also help them. We can help with documentation — although this has been a contentious issue — but at the least we can provide technical support. We can help them validate their science. And Ayurveda can help Allopathy in rediscovering the art of medicine as against the science of medicine. And by the same token, we can provide and restore the science of Alternative Medicine to the art of Alternative Medicine, which Ayurvedic practitioners are generally good at.

Therefore, I would say let us collaborate, let us shake hands and come together under a common umbrella, but not become one. If we do that, we will be helping each other take care of our deficiencies, instead of gnawing at each other's good points. If we do that, we will work together for the betterment of each one of us, for each other's modalities of health delivery, and for the betterment of all humanity; and not only humanity, but the flora and fauna of planet earth.

Pramod Kumar: Dr O. P. Yadava perhaps represents a very welcome trend amongst Allopathic doctors who are willing to explore possibilities in TM and CAM. In fact, Michelji was recently telling me about a survey done in Israel, which showed that when Allopathic doctors had gone on strike for two weeks, death rates in Israel had come down drastically during this period (Siegel-Itzkovich 2000: 1561)! Jokes aside, I request *Vaidya* Dr Ram Manoharji to talk to us about the case for Ayurveda and other approaches to health care.

P. Ram Manohar: I would have thought Dr O. P. Yadava would be building a case against the use of CAM, but he happens to be one of those Allopathic doctors who actually uses CAM and traditional medicinal modalities. To that extent, he has already expressed what I wanted to express. So I think I'll try to put a few things in perspective, in terms of what Dr O. P. Yadava has said, and whatever we can both consider to be the desired goal.

I think we must look at ground realities: we have two models in front of us now — one is the kind of model that is emerging in countries like the United States, and the other in a country like India. In both countries, I think the interactions between conventional medicine and what we now understand as CAM/TM are heading towards slightly different directions. In the US, there is a tendency for more and more Allopathic practitioners to re-evaluate the TM and CAM modalities and try to integrate it into their own practice. And the goal seems to be to achieve what is now called Integrative Medicine. However, in countries like the US, only an MD is allowed to practice medicine, whereas in India, not only does conventional Allopathic medicine have legal sanction, but various other medical systems are also in practice. So I think, broadly, we have two models to look at from a very practical level, and it would be interesting to see how these are functioning and evolving, to find how we can facilitate this growth towards a more complete healthcare system.

There is a lot of interaction, cross-fertilisation, adoption of techniques from other systems of medicine taking place at present. In a country like India, it is shocking to note that 90 per cent of Ayurvedic physicians are also practising Allopathic medicine and there is a lot of experimentation going on. Although at one level we would like to talk about an ideal, there is a big gap between what we idealise and what is actually happening at the ground level. So it may be fruitful look at these two models: one in which there is an increasing trend of trying to evaluate and build evidence of components of TM/CAM therapies — I wouldn't say that it is always like that even in the United States; there are a lot of CAM practitioners emerging and practising independently, but I think the overall trend is moving towards the incorporation of TM/CAM therapies into conventional medicine — and on the other hand, we have the example of India, where although there is an official-level sanction for all kinds of medical systems, it is not well regulated. There are many overlaps, and even a lot of Allopathic practitioners are using drugs from Ayurveda and other TMs. These two models present a good reference point to see what is really happening, and then compare with the ideal that Dr O. P. Yadava has presented before us. I think that will give us some direction to see how we can take this forward.

Pramod Kumar: I would like to mention that the Arya Vaidya Pharmacy — and particularly Dr Ram Manohar — has been involved in setting up chairs of Ayurveda in many US universities. I would like to invite Dr Ramesh Bijlani to talk about Yoga at AIIMS, as an Indian case study.

Ramesh Bijlani: When, in 2000, I was instrumental in establishing the Integral Health Clinic at AIIMS, there were many concerned people who didn't know what was actually going to happen; how this institution, which had been devoted exclusively to the practice of scientific medicine, would now start the practice of some alternative system of medicine. The way it was introduced, in fact, was neither as an alternative system of medicine nor as complementary medicine, but just medicine. Because by the year 2000, we had enough evidence in scientific medicine to show that the conventional way of treating medicine as a physical mode of treatment in which the mind–body relationship could be ignored was no longer valid. We had mounting evidence that the new killers of mankind, such as high blood pressure, heart disease, diabetes, and cancer, are closely related to mental stress. The good news was that unlike the conventional thought that made us believe that self-healing is limited only to non-acute diseases like common cold and diarrhoea, we found that it operated in the case of chronic diseases as well. All that we needed to do to activate the self-healing mechanism in chronic diseases was to reverse the condition that led to these conditions; and those conditions, briefly, were inadequate physical activity, eating too much of the wrong type of food, mental stress, smoking, inadequate sleep, and so on.

Thus, if we reverse these conditions, we could start reversing chronic disease. To give a practical shape to this approach, we needed a system that could combine a good lifestyle with a potent method for overcoming mental stress. And this is how modern medicine has rediscovered ancient techniques like Yoga, which combines superb lifestyles with potent prescriptions for lasting mental peace.

So we were going to use Yoga as a tool in mind–body medicine, an approach to provide a good package that could reverse the factors which led to chronic diseases, in the hope that reversing them would both prevent and treat them. The reason for it being called Integral Health Clinic — which is easily confused with Integrated Medicine, and so on — was that we were going to look at the practice of medicine as something which would look at the totality of the being. That is how all those who have gone deeper into the work of Sri Aurobindo and the Mother have used the term Integral Medicine. Whether it is Integral Yoga, Integral Education, Integral Psychology, or Integral Health, 'integral' refers to the recognition of the totality of the being, which includes not just the body, mind and intellect, but also the soul.

To give this a practical shape, we designed a nine-day intervention programme in which people came to us for a few hours per day, and did not only the physical practices of Yoga, but also received some information on what Yoga is and how it can be brought into daily life, how it can be used for stress management, how to eat wisely and well, and so on. This, admittedly, is a very limited way of looking at Yoga, but it was inevitable since the project was on a large-scale and those who came to us came primarily for prevention or management of diseases. It could not be assumed that they were interested solely in spiritual growth. When you give it a practical shape, these are the compromises one has to make. But what was interesting was that even in this approach, where so little was being done — compared to the whole discipline of Yoga — we still had dramatic results. Within nine days, we found that in more than 100 persons whose data was analysed, there was statistically significant reduction in fasting plasma glucose and improvement in the lipid profile, and this was published in the Journal of CAM in 2005 (Bijlani et al. 2005: 267–74).

Then there were other studies on another set of patients in the same clinic, where we found an improvement in the subjective well-being, a reduction in stress whether measured as a trait or as a present state of anxiety, an improvement in the antioxidant status, and an improvement in the ratio of parasympathetic to the sympathetic tone as measured as heart-rate variability. We also did a Randomised Control Trial in the same clinic on bronchial asthma on 60 people who were divided into two randomised groups of 30 each, and we found that there was an improvement in both the subjective and measurable objective variables in respiratory functions in these persons.

Of course, the question that is always raised when you provide a package like this is: which out of the following components is responsible for the improvement? That really is a question that arises from the reductionist approach of modern medicine, but is not, properly speaking, applicable to a holistic system because each of these components contributes. And it is very difficult to separate the effect of each; if we try to separate them, we will probably find that each of them is effective, but all of them put together are more effective than the algebraic sum of each of these components. They all work together.

Even within the short period that I was there — for a period of five years from the establishment of this facility — we could do a considerable amount of work that documented the effects of Yoga; and this is in keeping with a large amount of other work of a similar type coming from all over the world in the past two decades.

Pramod Kumar: I am sure all of us recognise that given that Yoga is perhaps the most widely accepted alternative therapy today, the experiences of Dr Ramesh Bijlani and the case studies being done at AIIMS would serve as prototypes for similar experiments being done elsewhere. I will now call upon Dr Nisha Money to share her experiences of applying Yoga techniques in the medical care set-up in the United States.

Nisha Money: First of all, I would like to say that I agree with the way the previous speakers have elaborated a case for bringing in Complementary and Alternative Medicine into Allopathy, specifically in the US. This is something that myself and my colleague Dr Matthew Fritts have been trying to bring about in our own work in a non-confrontational way. I think it is mainly in areas where conventional Allopathy doesn't seem to work well that there is such a huge need to look at other treatments. Where conventional treatments are not as effective in curing illnesses, we need to look to the East to see if there are other ways that could complement our treatment modalities.

I am in an active duty position in the US air force. And as you probably know, we have faced some difficult situations because of the wars. There has been quite a fallout, emotionally and physically, from the war — repercussions of what happened in Afghanistan and Iraq. It has been mainly in the area of Post Traumatic Stress Disorder (PTSD); it is something that we are facing considerably as a pressing medical issue in the US, especially with our armed forces. So our conventional treatment modalities which use cognitive-based therapies or Selective Serotonin Reuptake Inhibitors (SSRI) or antidepressants for Post Trauma Stress Treatment (PTST) have been somewhat effective, but we've now decided that we need to look more into other types of treatment that will really complement what we are actually doing and be helpful to our troops. That is how we expanded into looking at Eastern practices and Yoga. More specifically, *Yoga Nidra* is the technique that we looked at to see if it would be helpful at the psychological level. We have created a pilot study at the Walter Reid Medical Center, which is based in Washington DC. We have put army soldiers through this programme that we created, and we trained them in *Yoga Nidra* to help out with their symptoms and PTST, and we actually found enough evidence for us to do Randomised Control Trials.

So what my colleagues and I have done is that we have put together a proposal for a Randomised Control Trial in *Yoga Nidra* specifically to help as an adjunct therapy for PTST. It has enabled us to reach the level of psychological help that was not being provided by conventional therapy, and also suggested that there is a spiritual approach to treatment; I think *Yoga Nidra* has really spoken to a lot of the soldiers in a way that has hit home. They have been empowered with a skill-set that they can take home, without being dependent on a provider to help them psychologically. That is something that's really been a wonderful outcome of our study carried out in the military. And now we are taking it forward to a bigger programme by substantiating it and validating it with evidence-based data by running a Randomised Clinical Trial with *Yoga Nidra*. This is the foremost reason that we are here today.

Pramod Kumar: I request Dr Mathew Fritts to share his own experiences and talk to us about issues and problems in authenticating complementary and alternative medicine.

Matthew Fritts: I would like to take a couple of minutes to talk about research on TM and CAM. First of all, about why it is necessary, and then some ideas on how it can be done effectively. I think research on TM and CAM can really be a catalyst for the integration that Dr Ram Manohar has spoken about, for different reasons and for both the models that Dr Manohar spoke of. When we talk about TM and CAM in the United States, research is necessary to establish firmly the effectiveness of these therapies. And the reason is not only to make sure we are providing effective medicine, but also to set the groundwork for bringing TM and CAM on an equal level with Allopathic medicine in terms of legal sanction, as well as regulatory and policy issues.

At the present time, it is certainly not on an equal level. There is a large disparity in insurance coverage as well as licensure situations in the US and other Western countries. But the situation in India is slightly different, and as such the need for research here is also different. Although it is undeniable that there is still a need for strong evidence based on terms of effectiveness, my sense is that the need for research in India is more for reasons of safety. Dr Ram Manohar mentioned that 90 per cent of Ayurvedic physicians use Allopathic medicines without receiving training in it, and without being licensed to prescribe Allopathic medicines. There is some use of traditional medicines by Allopathic physicians without the requisite training. Some issues about safety can be raised here: the usage of drugs (both Allopathic and Ayurvedic) by untrained practitioners, the actual components of these therapies, heavy metal content in some Ayurvedic medicines, and other issues related to safety, such as interactions between Traditional Medicine and Allopathic medicines. So this is a major reason for conducting research on TM and CAM here in India, as well as in the world. These are concerns that are relevant globally.

Besides these, another reason why we need to conduct research on TM and CAM is really to facilitate its dissemination worldwide. There is so much knowledge and wisdom that has been collected over thousands of years in these traditional medical systems, and it is a shame that it has not spread throughout the world. The rest of the world can benefit from this knowledge, especially with regard to chronic diseases and conditions for which Allopathy really does not have an answer. Those are my reasons for the need for research on TM and CAM.

I will just back up a bit to explain my background in research: for a number of years, I was with the US National Institutes for Health, which is the US government's medical research agency; I am now with a non-profit organisation called the Samueli Institute in the Washington DC area. So let me shift now to talk a little about some ideas on how effectively we can conduct research on TM and CAM.

Usually the Randomised Control Trial is considered the gold standard, and Michel Danino in his introductory references mentions the recent meta-analysis of Homeopathy that was conducted, which declared categorically that Homeopathy is ineffective and that no further research was necessary. Part of the reason for this sort of false, negative finding is the special model for validity: Randomised Clinical Trial is not always the most appropriate form of research for TM and CAM. There are a variety of other options. I do not have the time to go into all of the other options, but they range anywhere from qualitative research to observational methodologies, laboratory testing, etc. So, depending on the outcome that is needed, we need to be prudent in selecting an appropriate methodology, and do not always have to conform to the Western bio-medical view, in which the RCT is the gold standard.

The last thing I want to talk about concerns the levels of evidence that are required. Often, a lot of medical decision-making is done based on case reports and case series, which really are not a sufficient level of evidence to be making policy decisions on, at national levels, or even at local levels affecting thousands of people. So, one of the things that Samueli Institute wants to do is build the evidence base at a higher level, working up from lower evidence levels — from case reports and case series, to conducting trials which may not necessarily be randomised and controlled, and then ultimately synthesising the results of individual studies into meta-analysis and systematic reviews, which would be an appropriate level of evidence on which to make policy and legal decisions at a national, and ultimately at a global level. These are some thoughts on how research can be a catalyst and vector for the necessary integration of TM and CAM therapies with that of Allopathic medicine.

Makarand R. Paranjape: On this issue of integration, may I add something? I think the approach varies from country to country, or from civilisation to civilisation. In Brazil, for instance, there are many Allopathic doctors who also study and bring in CAM. They say it helps the patients and also helps them grow as healing practitioners. In Singapore, the two systems do not mix, but even if they are kept separate, both are used. So there are many possibilities here.

Pramod Kumar: Thank you for having joined us in this discussion. I now request Dr Sujatha to explain the social implications of TM and CAM.

V. Sujatha: Ayurveda's view of the body and its ways, and methods of trying to treat the body of illness, are different. Is there any ground or possibility for a dialogue between two different ways of looking at the human body? This is the issue at stake here. The question is not whether a dialogue is possible, but what the terms of the dialogue are. You see, often by way of dialogue, syncretism, integration, what is happening is that the indigenous systems are made to translate their own categories and terms in the language of another system. Dialogue has happened between different medical systems earlier in history. Siddha and Ayurveda have interacted. There has been a lot of interaction between Siddha and the Chinese system of medicine, where many basic ideas of eye diseases, that is, Ophthalmology, have gone back and forth. There has been an exchange between Greek medicine and Unani, and Unani and Ayurveda. So systems of medicine have interacted earlier. The point is in the earlier situation, every system of medicine could retain its own integrity, its own *svabhava* (nature), and assimilate or selectively assimilate from other systems according to its own terms and needs. But this is not the case with bio-medicine, which was introduced in India during colonial rule under enormous pressure.

There was a deliberate attempt to discriminate against indigenous practices and suppress them. This was the condition of interaction between bio-medicine and Ayurveda. Unlike earlier interactions between other modalities within the indigenous systems, the interaction between Ayurveda and bio-medicine is not characterised by mutuality. There is no give and take. The most charitable statement that has been made is that bio-medicine is open, but will only take peripheral aspects like empathy and care from Ayurveda; it has nothing to learn with regard to science, that is, the science of the body. Ayurveda, on the other hand, can take science and methods of verification from Allopathy. This is the most open position on the interaction at present. This is the level of mutuality envisaged. This is also where the problem lies in all the debates about dialogues. What are the terms of the dialogue and who dictates those terms?

This brings me to one of the most important points being raised: the Randomised Controlled Trial. Before we raise the question of whether Randomised Controlled Trials can be applied to Ayurvedic medicine, my question is, are they even adequate for Allopathic medicine? For instance, within Allopathic medicine, within the philosophy of science and among Allopathic practitioners, there is a very big debate about the RCT: you develop a drug in a laboratory and then RCTs are conducted for a few years, in which the drug is tested on a population of 8,000, and then is made available throughout the world. Is this a sufficient way of testing a medicine before making it available to the public at large? Although the drug may specify the side-effects and everything might be stated, the doctors do not hold any ethical responsibility for adverse consequences of the drug. This is evident from the fact that a very high percentage of deaths, even in the established medical school hospitals in the US, are caused by what they call iatrogenic diseases, that is, diseases or deaths caused by the medicine or the surgery itself. Can you think of a system killing its own patients, not intentionally, but killing them nonetheless? So this is the crisis even within Allopathy, which is voiced by a fraternity of medical doctors. When this technique is debated even within its own system, how can we recommend it to a holistic system like Ayurveda? This is something that Ayurvedic practitioners who strongly canvass for RCTs should deeply consider.

Lastly, I wish to conclude by answering the question raised here as to what is the most appropriate model for a country like India — whether it is what mainstream bio-medicine calls the 'CAM' model of integration, which we have just spoken about, or whether it should be another model. I would think this so-called 'CAM' model, that is, the model by which you validate in the laboratory the so-called alternative systems within the bio-medical framework, will lead to a homogenous world where Ayurveda will inherit the problems of bio-medicine. What is the idea behind having many systems? What is the true idea of pluralism? Is it not that one system should offset the limitations of the other so that people have more options? If you want to mould Ayurveda in the same way, such that in two different rooms two professionals would be sitting, where one man will give a pill, while the other gives a herbal drug — this is reducing Ayurveda to a herbal adjunct. If we follow this model, very soon Ayurveda will become a herbal appendage to bio-medicine, and will only be found in spas, in medical tourism such as Pancha Karma medical tourism, while bio-medicine will inhabit the hospitals, as it has done in Europe.

Two hundred years ago, in Europe, the mainstream medicine was Naturopathy, Hydrotherapy, Homeopathy, and other therapies. Bio-medicine was at the periphery, or it was an alternative. But within 200 years, it has occupied the hospitals, and these holistic therapies are relegated to the spa and the beauty salons. This is what will happen in

India, too. On the other hand, where is the question of validation? I will conclude with this one point. The point is that each medical system may have a dialogue with another, but each system should retain its own integrity; it should have its own methods of verification and the validity of its medicines — how effective its medicines are should be determined in actual problem-solving.

In this respect, I would like to draw your attention to a programme by the Tamil Nadu government, where Ayurveda was applied in public health to solve the problem of iron malnutrition among pregnant mothers and young women. It has been successfully working within the health infrastructure to solve the public health problem of anaemia, entirely from the point of view of Ayurveda. Due to a paucity of time, I cannot elaborate on this (for a complete report, see Girija et al. 2005). But the point is that the validity of Ayurveda need not be determined in the laboratory. It can be determined in its ability to actually solve the problems in front of people.

Pramod Kumar: Thank you, Dr Sujatha, for cautioning us about the consequences of trying to force TM and CAM into the framework of bio-medicine or conventional medicine. In fact, this issue is relevant not only in the context of healing, but also in all dialogues of science and spirituality. This is what Dharampal also points out — that all studies of native societies, whether it be of their traditional medicine or their traditional science, is always done through the colonial framework or from the conqueror's perspective. This is something that will not serve the purpose at all. Thank you, again. Lastly, I call upon Professor Makarand R. Paranjape to deliberate on the key issues of how we understand spirituality in the context of healing.

Makarand R. Paranjape: When we were planning this conference, it was our earnest wish to encourage dialogue between two seemingly different systems of medicine: traditional medical practices — what they call CAM practices — and what is now clearly the dominant system of bio-medicine; and bio-medicine has become not just dominant and dominating, but something that's going to take over even the plural space of India, as Dr Sujatha has pointed out.

Let me focus on two things. The first — what do we mean by spirituality? I think that one way of defining it would be the recognition and the action of the non-corporeal portion of our being. What do I mean by non-corporeal? Well, basically, it refers to something beyond or more than the body. Now, of course, what the body in itself is, is a mystery. The body can be more than itself. For instance, there is a view that we have three bodies — the physical (*sthula*), the subtle (*sukshma*) and causal (*karana*). No wonder, it is even more complicated when we use words like trans-physicality. When we don't fully understand physicality, that's when we introduce terms like trans-physicality. Maybe there is just this *one* body, of which the physical, emotional, intellectual, and beyond that, the spiritual aspects, are all part. Or, as Sri Ramana Maharashi used to say, even the body is merely a thought, *vichara*, as is the world. We do not know. We have to think about these things carefully. But non-corporeal means going back to the original understanding of spirituality. There is a body which dies when we die, but there is another portion of us which does not die and that is called the spirit. Recognition means acknowledging that there is such an entity, there is such an aspect to our selves that is beyond our body. And action means to do something about it, perhaps through a daily practice — it could be a prayer, it could be a *mantra*, it could be chanting, it could be meditation. So, if we understand spirituality as the recognition and action of the non-corporeal part of our being, then the question arises — what role does it play in healing?

From our two-and-a-half days of deliberation, it is very clear that it plays a very important role in at least two different ways. The first is preventive, as Dr Bijlani has shown us. Most of the diseases that kill people today are caused by what we might call erroneous or self-destructive lifestyles. The moment you introduce spirituality into a person's lifestyle, we find a dramatic improvement in the quality of life. This is because even if you take a well-documented programme like Sri Sri Ravishankar's Sudharshan Kriya, one of the first effects of the Sudharshan Kriya is that intoxicating habits are reduced. And almost everybody that I know personally who has taken to any spiritual path has found a remarkable reduction in, say, tobacco addiction, alcoholism, or any other kind of addiction. So spirituality plays a part in changing the lifestyle of the people who practice it, and this is true, as we all know, of yoga. Now, if you change the lifestyle of someone, then the chances of illness or falling into self-destructive patterns of disease are reduced by a reduction in stress and in poisonous habits. So the disease is reduced. So spirituality plays a very important preventive role.

However, I might add that it also plays a curative role. How? This can be explained if you think of Ayurveda itself as a spiritual practice, because in Ayurveda, there is no split, as I understand it from experts, between the science and the spirituality. Both must go hand-in-hand — in fact this split, epistemologically even in the West, is only 200 years old. So it is not necessarily something eternal or God-given. From this perspective, spirituality can play a curative role too. I am not counting here the role played by intercessory prayer, pranic healing, and other non-material methods.

So it plays a preventive role, it plays a curative role, and finally, spirituality also plays a palliative role. That is, when you cannot decrease the pain, or a patient is terminally ill, when people are dying of a disease that is not curable, then spirituality alleviates suffering. It prepares people for death. It prepares people, perhaps for an after-life. It helps them cope with the pain, and thereby reduces suffering. Victor Frankl, quoting Nietzsche, said: 'He who has a *why* to live for can bear with almost any *how*' (1985: 12). In other words, that which causes suffering is not just pain, but pain which has no explanation, pain which does not have reason, pain which is arbitrary, accidental, and meaningless. That causes incredible cognitive trauma. But the moment pain is put into perspective, people find that they have relief. So in all three ways, spirituality plays a very important role in healing.

I want to end by saying that often, we make a distinction between the East and the West, and sometimes between modernity and tradition, but I think we need to see increasingly how they are not intrinsically or necessarily or automatically opposed to one another. And to see how, either indirectly or directly, despite this duality that we construct — even if it is heuristic, even if it is strategic, even if it is for purposes of argument — we may find different strategies for making similar points. In our discussion, we saw that the fundamental idea of what health means in our tradition is *svasthya,* that is, our own *sva* (natural self) + *avastha* (state of being), that is, our own natural state of being. But if you look at what health has come to mean in modern terms, people tend to think that it is just the absence of disease. If we go back to the original meaning, then health means to be whole. To be healthy is to be whole and to be whole is also to be whole. So, there is no dichotomy.

Pramod Kumar: Thank you Makarandji. Organisers always keep their best speakers for the last.

We will now open the session for interaction. If you have any questions for any of the panellists, you can introduce yourself and mention the name of the panellist that you wish to address the question to. If it is a general question, you can just ask it, and then perhaps one of the panellists could respond to it. Over to the audience: any questions?

Questioner 1: I am an Engineering student. This is a general question addressed to the doctors of Allopathic medicine present here: what is your opinion on the efficacy of alternative healing systems?

O. P. Yadava: Well, I think there is definitely awareness among the Allopathic physicians about the limitations of Allopathy. That is the reason we are entering this dialogue, which we had not done till, say, five to ten years ago. And that itself I think is a great advancement. If we at least know what we don't know, then I think we will do well enough. And Allopathic practitioners are beginning to realise their limitations. At this moment, most people are using alternative medicine or referring patients to alternative medicine for end-of-life issues — terminal heart failure, terminal cancers. But they do not seem to recognise the uses of alternative medicine at an earlier stage. Also, most people in Allopathy are beginning to realise the role of alternative medicine in prevention and prophylaxis; but the majority of doctors dealing with the middle range of early to mid-stage disease are not willing to accept the advantages of alternative medicine.

Nisha Money: I can provide an answer from the Western perspective, specifically the US. A lot of us there in the Allopathy-trained world would be more open to alternatives when there is evidence-based data driving the Complementary and Alternative modalities. And those of us keen on incorporating it are also interested in the research component of it. We are also realising, especially right now, the widespread occurrence in the US of the public seeking these treatments and paying out of their own pocket for it. What we would like to have is (*a*) greater regulation, and (*b*) we would want to know if there are any kind of drug interactions that happen with the herbal products that people are taking, which they are not openly confiding about to their mainstream healthcare providers; they may be taking other drugs or herbs that could actually be counter-productive to some of the medications that they are taking. In addition to these couple of reasons — safety and the possibility of expanding treatments for individuals — I can say the great emphasis in the US these days is that we seem to recognise that we are not addressing the spiritual component of the healing process. A lot of us who are becoming more sympathetic to mental health issues and psychosomatic issues are really coming into this awareness — that we need to hit the dimension or actually access the dimension of an individual's spiritual nature.

Questioner 2: I am Tom McKenzie from Global Perspectives on Science and Spirituality, Paris. I am just having a little bit of difficulty understanding what you just meant by 'spirituality'. Makarand, if I understand correctly, I think what you understand by spirituality is really just leading a healthy and balanced lifestyle. And to a certain extent, what Ayurveda is providing is a sort of whole conceptual framework for basically leading a healthy life. As far as I am concerned, that absolutely seems fine, and I cannot imagine any sort of doctor in his right mind having any objection to this sort of concept of spirituality. I think we possibly get into more difficult territory when trying to find spirituality as, for instance, intercessory prayer. People did mention this; it was brought up earlier. Is this perceived as a problem here? As far as you are concerned, are you defining spirituality as a healthy way of life, or does it go into these other definitions as well?

Makarand R. Paranjape: You know, one of the doctors who was there, Dr B. M. Hegde, the former Vice-Chancellor of Manipal Medical University, defined spirituality as just sharing and caring. This is not what I meant when I said spirituality is the recognition and action that derives from, or that arises from, the acceptance of a non-corporeal part of one's being. That is, not simply leading a healthy lifestyle, but a recognition that we are more than just our physical bodies and it may have many implications, including intercession and prayer. I think this is what Dr Moody meant, especially in the context of mental health and psychiatric treatment. There, certainly, meditation, prayer, or any other way of reaching something larger than us, seems to have a definite role. On the other hand, when we are treating other diseases, prayer and so on may be supplementary, not substitutive, of regular treatment. In Ayurveda, too, other lines of treatment, including prayer, *japa*, even astrology, are seen as useful supplements. The idea is to address the totality — or at any rate, as much of it as we might access — in the process of healing. Right here, in the Arya Veda Pharmacy Hospital, for instance, there is a temple to Dhanvantri, the god of healing. Rituals and rites are regularly performed here.

Regarding prayer, there are studies to show how apparently prayer can help in healing. There are also studies to show that prayer does not help at all, as some were quoting. And similarly, there are studies to show that to some extent, *mantra*s are capable of healing. Even if this were a placebo effect, why rule it out if it helps? There are also practical examples. For example, Sujatha was talking about how she witnessed the treatment of snake bite. The healer used a combination of mantras, plus 64 herbs. Now what worked, we do not know. It did work, though, because the patient recovered.

So my point is that these things, which are considered problematic by the scientific community, have still not been abandoned by the common people, especially if they are perceived to work. We cannot entirely banish 'magic' from our midst. That is why I don't think that spirituality is only leading a healthy lifestyle, or it is only caring and sharing, although both may be outcomes of it.

Spirituality, then, is a recognition that we are not merely our bodies, it is the recognition of the 'spirit' or the 'self' which is non-corporeal. Now this may have deep and far-reaching implications on one's life. It may lead to a definite soteriology or teleology, or simply to what some people call self-realisation. Of course, some people talk about other entities like the divine and God. So for me, all of those things are a part of spirituality, and I think that when it comes to healing, that is one area where even sceptics seem to give some credit to how these 'non-scientific' things help. I am told that more and more hospitals in the United States not only have a chaplain or somebody available to help a patient spiritually, but they also do not forbid patients from trying out other therapies in addition to the regular treatment that is going on. Regardless of whether they believe these things work or not, they say there is no harm if the patient feels better. And Dr Yadava was telling me that while preparing a patient's case history when s/he is admitted, her/his belief systems are noted down in great detail and respected, by saying that we may not share them, but if that is going to affect their state of mind and lead to a faster cure or better recovery, then so be it.

So what I am trying to say is that even without accepting the alternative therapies or CAM or traditional medicine in totality, or accepting their epistemological foundations, a lot of modern medicine has started recognising their utility. That is why, when we return to what Sujatha was saying about the terms of interaction, of course we must admit they are very unfair. But you know, sometimes victories do not have to be trumpeted. There can be very quiet victories. There can be slow changes and shifts which are so significant that without pushing matters into, should I say, a confrontation, a lot is still happening and can be gained from.

As to challenging the primacy of the multinationals and how they are taking over Ayurveda and changing it, these are things we should concentrate on in India, because we have a deep interest in this.

The last thing I wanted to say is that unfortunately, we find this reverse trend: abroad, in the so-called advanced societies, there is much greater openness to CAM, TM, and other therapies, while here in India, more and more poor people, even people leading traditional lifestyles, ask for an injection when they visit an Ayurvedic doctor. So a labourer comes in with a pain and all he says is, 'Doctor, give me an injection'. So poorer people are moving towards Allopathy in India and the rich people, imitating the West, are going for Reiki and Pranic healing, and all that. I think, from an Indian point of view, we need to address some of these issues, and educate people that traditional methods are not so bad, after all.

Pramod Kumar: Dr O. P. Yadava, would you like to add something?

O. P. Yadava: Regarding spirituality: this question has been asked so many times. Sorry, I don't quite understand what spirituality is myself, and I think perhaps this question should be answered by some realised master and not by ordinary mortals like us. If I really look around and ask, 'Can I recognise any person whom I can truly call spiritual?' then I fail to do so. But if you look at every child, you find spirituality in every child. A child does everything wrong: s/he breaks things, s/he eats wrong, wets the bed, everything . . . What is there in the child that is so adorable? That is spirituality. What is it? I do not know. To me, that is spirituality.

Makarand R. Paranjape: Well-said; innocence or guilelessness is certainly one mark of spirituality, but as Dr Yadava himself said, self-mastery, or realisation, is another. In the light of cold hard reason, these qualities cannot be quantified or proven, of course. But even many scientists try to realise themselves as human beings, and try to live integrated and happy lives.

Pramod Kumar: Any other questions?

Questioner 3: I am Dr Rama Jayasundar. I was trained at AIIMS in New Delhi, but am now researching Ayurveda and Quantum Physics. I have two questions and I would like Dr Ram Manohar and Dr Yadava to answer them. There is so much talk about standardisation and scientific validation. If you can both tell me what exactly it is, and what the aim of that standardisation is? Is it standardisation like Allopathic medicine for active ingredients? I would like to hear from Dr Ram Manohar first, because he is an Ayurvedic *vaidya*, and then from Dr Yadava, and I would also like them to answer the question about scientific validation.

P. Ram Manohar: I think if you look at Ayurveda as a knowledge system, even within the tradition there is this notion of validation. Knowledge has to be *prama*; it has to be measured and confirmed. But then this demand for scientific validation in clinical medicine is something different, as Dr Sujatha was pointing out. It is a different kind of validation which you are forced to conform to. Ayurveda is not against validation. But the whole issue is that the Western, I mean, the scientific model of validation is not the only way to validate knowledge. So I think it's very important — as in our example, where we have been involved in a clinical research programme with some US universities, and it has created an opportunity for us to engage in a dialogue. We ventured to do this because of the belief that Ayurveda is a knowledge system, and that we are not against validation. I mean, we need not shy away from that. But we also understood that we need to enter into a dialogue — as we have with mutual respect — and try to evolve a more satisfactory methodology. The whole issue is communication. I mean at a deeper level, it's just that; people speaking two different languages are trying to understand what is happening in that situation. There is no time to go into all the details. But when we had this interaction with scientists from the US, they said that as long as it fits into what they considered some basic points that they wished to conform to, it was perfectly okay with them. We said we could not compromise on some principles of Ayurveda. So if we could come to a common platform of understanding, then it was perfectly all right from both sides. What we achieved is a unique design of a Randomised Clinical Trial.

You know that in classical conventional research, you have one particular drug which you test against one particular condition, and you have the same drug being administered throughout the clinical trial. But we have entered a clinical trial design with the UCLA with a conventional rheumatologist who is very well known in the US, and we have done this with support from the NIH. In our trial, we are studying Ayurveda as a whole. I do not think there has been a clinical trial where the physician, that is, the Ayurvedic physician, has had complete freedom to diagnose every patient. Michelji was talking about individualised treatment. Every patient in our trial is given a different combination of medicines and every time the patient visits, the physician changes the medicine. We think that if there is a very serious dialogue between scientists and Ayurvedic physicians, we can bring this issue of validation to a higher plane. Ultimately, I think validation is necessary, because otherwise we cannot consider Ayurveda a knowledge system.

Rama Jayasundar: Is this synonymous with documentation?

P. Ram Manohar: What do you mean by documentation?

Rama Jayasundar: By documentation, I mean that whatever procedures the *vaidya* follows should be documented, and their results verified.

P. Ram Manohar: Yes, I mean, you are talking about observational studies?

Rama Jayasundar: Yes.

O. P. Yadava: Documentation is an integral part of validation. Now let me get to your first question about controlled trials, and so forth. There are certain physical parameters and I am sure there will be certain trans-physical and metaphysical parameters. Certainly, modern technology can document those physical parameters. We cannot document the non-physical parameters. So the terms of reference for these trials should be provided by the alternative medicine providers. They should not be dogmatic about refusing scientific scrutiny. But the terms of reference should be provided by them. I give you a simple example. You say a particular drug works for blood pressure. What is the difficulty in subjecting 100 patients to observation, recording their blood pressure before the drug is given, and then recording their blood pressure afterwards? There should be no problem? This is a simple model.

Rama Jayasundar: So, it is a simple documentation.

O. P. Yadava: This debate has been raging for a while. A lot of what is considered documentation is merely technology — some sort of gadget or machine recording data. Of course, this is just ignorance. If a system has been in use and has worked for thousands of years, surely that is a sort of documentation too. So actually, what we have offered is something tremendous and phenomenal.

You saw today that we were debating whether Transcendental Meditation works or not. And Swami Nithyananda's programme — they showed the brain scans before and after to prove decreased brain activity and a state of calm. Now that is documentation and validation.

So I ask, why don't you subject yourselves to validation? After all, science is ultimately about this. And it is common to both Allopathy and Ayurveda. It is not that the science for Allopathy is different for Ayurveda like it is for, say, normal mechanics and quantum mechanics.

How is it that we are unable to document the very simple fact that alternative medicine is based on science? That is my problem, speaking from within Allopathy — that you are not allowing documentation and validation, without which I find it difficult to accept it. But I am convinced personally that, alternative medicine itself being a science, if given the opportunity, can come out with flying colours. Please do not be scared. Subject yourselves. You will succeed. But you are resisting.

Rama Jayasundar: I personally do not resist. For the benefit of the audience, I am a physicist by training and profession. But right now I am studying Ayurveda. So I am an Ayurvedic doctor as well. Of course, my initial reason for entering Ayurveda when I was 40-plus was that I was interested in scientific validation and standardisation. Those are the words I heard most commonly when it came to criticising Ayurveda. I am also a faculty member at AIIMS. And there are many groups in AIIMS working in and doing research on Ayurveda. In fact, I will take a couple of minutes to explain my position so that things are put in perspective. When I approached my Institute Director for permission to do this five-and-a-half years' course, he said, 'you are really crazy to want to do this, to go through five-and-a-half years of an undergraduate medical course at your age of 41'. I was at the peak of my career at that time. He said, 'you know you don't have to go through this five-and-a-half years' course to do research in Ayurveda'. But I said, if I wanted to do research in Physics, I should study Physics. Applying the same logic, I should study Ayurveda to do research in Ayurveda. So I entered the field with all these ideas — that my contribution to Ayurveda will be scientific validation and standardisation. Having gone through the course, I do not claim to be an expert in Ayurveda, but at least I know what to do and what not to do. So documentation is certainly something that has to be done; it is the need of the hour. There is absolutely no doubt about it. And I don't think there is a lot of resistance from the Ayurvedic community. Maybe Dr Ram Manohar would be in a better position to speak about this, because he has more experience.

P. Ram Manohar: Just to clarify, let me speak from my own experience. We had a study sponsored by the WHO. It was conducted 25 years ago. And I think this will illustrate the basic difference. As Dr O. P. Yadava said, some kind of validation and documentation is essential for any knowledge system to be promoted, but it is the approach that is crucial. The study should be designed in such a way that it is an effective test.

So there was this WHO study, conducted over a seven-year study period. But in the end, it concluded that Ayurveda does not have any effect. Whatever effect Ayurveda has is not even as good as the equivalent of an aspirin.

That was 25 years ago. During all this time, these findings and files were shelved. Then a few scientists from the US came and dug up these files. They surprisingly found that the outcomes were actually encouraging. The patients had improved with the treatment. And yet the conclusion was that Ayurveda does not have any drug that is the equivalent of aspirin.

This is what I mean when I say that the entire design is important. When the WHO study was conducted, the whole idea was to see that Allopathic doctors of India were involved. These doctors from ICMR (Indian Council of Medical Research) were only interested to see if they could discover some herb or some combination which they could use in their own practice.

That was not possible because Ayurvedic physicians here gave so many medicines that the ICMR doctors found it absolutely confounding, and they could not understand what was happening. The patient gets an oil massage, after five days he gets another *kashayam*, then he gets a powder, then something else — you know, it was not something that could be replicated in the Allopathic model. So they concluded that not a single drug could be isolated to show predictable effects.

But 25 years later, almost miraculously, the real results surfaced. The very same tests, on further scrutiny, were actually shown to have worked quite well, in that most patients had recovered, or done much better after the treatment.

That is why we believe in truth. I think if we wait, truth will ultimately be discovered.

Interestingly, it was this WHO study which eventually helped us to design and modify the clinical trial design.

Dr Daniel E. Furst from UCLA, who had elaborate interactions with us, listened as we explained all the problems and situations, and he said there was absolutely nothing wrong in looking at the effect of the entire process, the whole Ayurvedic system, instead of trying to isolate one drug which would prove one result.

So I am sure if we have doctors like Dr O. P. Yadava collaborating and helping us, instead of those ICMR doctors, we would have no difficulties.

We tried a lot to get local rheumatologists to participate in our study, which we were doing for the National Institute of Health (NIH), USA. The rheumatologists said they were not interested in promoting superstition. This is the feedback that we received in Coimbatore and in Kerala. Here, our experience is that doctors from the West were actually much more open. They were willing to even modify that which is considered the gold standard, something which cannot be manipulated at all. Dr Furst was willing to say okay, you give whatever medicines you want, I just want to look at the outcomes. So we could still bring in science, as well as traditional perspectives. If we converge on equal terms, I think we can take this issue of validation to a higher plane, and then accord respectability to Ayurveda as a knowledge system.

Pramod Kumar: Any more questions?

Questioner 4: As a student of medicine, I have heard all that was said in the past one hour. I am unclear about something; it would be helpful if you could tell me what exactly you mean by integration. Is it like, if someone has a disease or a problem, they must go to an Allopath, a *vaidya,* and then arrive at a consensus? Is that how you understand integration? Also, if we look at the actual situation, especially in rural areas where people lack basic medical facilities, how we can apply all this there?

P. Ram Manohar: I think this is what I was trying to say. I do not know whether I could express it very clearly. I said that we must relate to ground realities. I mean, it is very difficult to integrate. There is one model in the US, it goes through the screening process where you try to build evidence, and then it is mainstreamed and becomes much more visible. But in a country like India, where we have multiple medical systems and so much heterogeneity even from a social point of view, it does create a lot of problems. I am not sure what the answers are. I think we need to have greater transparency. How this can be brought about is not very clear at the moment. There has to be a lot of interaction between medical practitioners of various medical systems. Even a system like Ayurveda is very heterogeneous. The way it is practised in south India is different from the way it is practiced in north India. So our ancient people, they tried one solution — but since it was so confusing, they would consult an astrologer to find out which physician they must go to! I do not know whether that is the situation we are in now. It is really very difficult to find out who is the best physician, which is the best medical system for you. And that's what I really wanted to point out. I think we need to look at these social implications.

Pramod Kumar: Dr Ramesh Bijlani, would you like to say something on this?

Ramesh Bijlani: Well, I think the most important thing is what system you believe in. Because in medicine, nothing works with everybody, and something works with at least somebody. If you have faith in something, that itself will be a very important factor in your recovery. And I think we have enough scientific evidence for that now: in most diseases, the evidence proves that the hero, in fact, is the body itself. Which means your body's own wisdom is quite capable of recovery, and what physicians can do at the most is assist the self-healing mechanisms in different ways. That is something that physicians can do irrespective of the system, and provided you have faith in the system, the chances are that you will do well.

Pramod Kumar: Dr Sujatha, would you like to say something?

V. Sujatha: With regard to your question about what the patient is supposed to do, generally studies show that Indian patients are very good at making judgements. I am a sociologist. When we visited some of the interior regions in central Tamil Nadu, we found that even the average villager, who is not so educated, uses allopathic medicine when he has a fever and wants instant relief because he has to go to work the next day. When he has a runny nose, he used an Ayurvedic fomentation. So they have good judgement. Even women go for delivery to the hospital, but they are notorious for non-compliance. They do not take the tonics given for the infants, but breastfeed them. Then these people also say that for them, Allopathy is associated with curative functions — *nalla irukka pillaikku poi ivalo periya oosiya* (why insert such a huge needle into a baby who is doing well). So they have their own rationale and an idea of how different medical systems are. They have their *vaidya*. And then they have the doctor. In fact, this has been an entire field of study — how people take decisions. It is expected that you will be wiser than any one of the service providers in choosing the most suitable medical framework for your condition.

I think we would like to preserve this autonomy. We should not allow any system to say you should use only this or that. We should respect the patients' right to choose, and preserve the pluralism of medical systems and practices in our country.

Pramod Kumar: On that note, I bring this panel discussion to a close, thanking each and every one of the panelists and all of you in the audience.

Notes

1. This session was recorded before a live audience at Amrita Viswavidyalaya, Coimbatore. On the last day of the three-day conference on 'The Science and Spirituality of Healing', 15–17 February 2008, the participants travelled from Arsha Vidya Gurukulam in Annakatti to the university to share their final outcome with an invited audience of students and teachers from Amrita Viswavidyalaya.
2. This edited transcript of the concluding panel discussion at the conference is meant to complement the opening face-off between modern bio-sciences, as represented by Dr Pushpa Mitra Bhargava, and alternative therapeutics, on whose behalf the Ayurvedic practitioner and researcher, Dr Ram Manohar, spoke. What we observe in the opening dialogue is an example of incommensurable views, mostly because of the 'hard' scientific position assumed by Dr Bhargava. In this panel discussion, however, we have multiple points of view, from those who are votaries of modern science and those who work in other disciplines. Instead of a stark opposition, we now notice a plurality that is enabling when it comes to the healing arts. Our attempt was to capture this pluralism in a multiplicity of actual voices, rather than summarise their positions and collapse the polyphony that modern scientific discourse discourages. Perhaps such a humanistic and dialogic 'conclusion' is only appropriate in a debate that has a long way to go.

References

Bijlani, R. L., R. P. Vempati, R. K. Yadav, R. B. Ray, V. Gupta, R. Sharma, N. Mehta, and S. C. Mahapatra. 2005. 'A Brief but Comprehensive Lifestyle Education Program Based on Yoga Reduces Risk Factors for Cardiovascular Disease and Diabetes Mellitus', *Journal of Alternative and Complementary Medicine*, 11 (2): 267–74.

Frankl, Victor Emil. 1985. *Man's Search for Meaning*. New York: Washington Square Press.

Girija, P. L. T., T. M. Mukundan, L. Ranganathan, and T. M. Srinivasan (eds). 2005. 'Editorial', *Saneevani Ayurveda Foundation Newsletter*, 3. Available online at http://www.samanvaya.com/main/contentframes/knowledge/articles/pdfs/october.PDF (accessed 5 November 2011).

Shang, A., K. Huwiler-Müntener, L. Nartey, P. Jüni, S. Dörig, J. A. Sterne, D. Pewsner, and M. Egger. 2005. 'Are the Clinical Effects of Homoeopathy Placebo Effects? Comparative Study of Placebo-Controlled Trials of Homoeopathy and Allopathy', *Lancet*, 366 (9487): 726–32.
Siegel-Itzkovich, Judy. 2000. 'Doctors' Strike in Israel May Be Good For Health', *British Medical Journal*, 320 (1561): 1561.

About the Editor

Makarand R. Paranjape is Chairperson and Professor of English at Centre for English Studies, School of Language, Literature and Culture Studies, Jawaharlal Nehru University, New Delhi. He served as the inaugural Indian Council for Cultural Relations (ICCR) Chair in Indian Studies at the National University of Singapore (2010–11). His recent publications include *The Death and Afterlife of Mahatma Gandhi* (2014), *Making India: Colonialism, National Culture, and the Afterlife of Indian English Authority* (2013), *Another Canon: Indian Texts and Traditions in English* (2010), and *Altered Destinations: Self, Society and Nation in India* (2009). He is also the Principal Investigator of an international project on 'Science and Spirituality in India'.

Notes on Contributors and Discussants

Pushpa Mittra Bhargava was the founder-director of the Centre for Cellular and Molecular Biology (CCMB) and a recipient of the prestigious Padma Bhushan award. His recent publications (with Chandana Chakrabarty) include *The Saga of Indian Science Since Independence in a Nutshell* (2003) and *Angels, Devil and Science: A Collection of Articles on Scientific Temper* (2007).

Ramesh Bijlani is currently a Trustee of Sri Aurobindo Ashram-Delhi Branch. He was the founder of the Integral Health Clinic, Department of Physiology, All India Institute of Medical Sciences (AIIMS), New Delhi, where he served as Professor and Head of Physiology for many years. His recent publications include *Back to Health through Yoga* (2008) and *Medical Research: All you wanted to know but did not know whom to ask* (2008).

Suhita Chopra Chatterjee is a Professor at the Department of Humanities and Social Sciences, Indian Institute of Technology, Kharagpur (IIT-K). Her publications include *Discourses on Aging and Dying* (with Priyadarshi Patnaik and Vijayaraghavan M. Chariar, 2008), and 'Palliative Care in India: Ethical Issues Underlying Paradigmatic Shifts', *Eubios Journal of Asian and International Bioethics* 17 (4, 2007).

Michel Danino, author, educationist and scholar, is the Convener of the International Forum for India's Heritage. Living in India since 1997, he has lectured widely at several cultural and educational institutions on aspects of Indian civilisation. His recent publications include *Indian Culture and India's Future* (2011) and *The Lost River: On the Trail of the Sarasvati* (2010).

Matthew Fritts is a Clinical Research Associate at the Samueli Institute, Virginia, USA. He has more than a decade of experience in research on complementary and integrative medicine (CAM), including four years at the National Institutes of Health. His primary research areas are mind–body interventions for chronic and mental illness, and traditional medical systems for HIV/AIDS.

Rama Jayasundar holds a Ph.D. in Physics (Nuclear Magnetic Resonance or NMR) from Cambridge University, UK. Apart from her main training as a physicist, she completed a five-and-a-half years' Ayurvedic medical course from Chennai in 2008. She is currently with the Department of NMR, All India Institute of Medical Sciences (AIIMS), New Delhi. In 2002, she became the first Indian to be invited to chair scientific sessions at the Conference of International Society for Magnetic Resonance in Medicine, USA.

Pramod Kumar was educated at Indian Institute of Technology, Madras (IIT-M) and soon thereafter joined the Amrita Viswavidyalaya as a teacher. He has been active in promoting the study of Indian knowledge systems in conventional engineering curricula.

P. Ram Manohar is an Ayurvedic physician by training and currently the Director of Research, Arya Vaidya Pharmacy, Coimbatore. He has authored research papers on Ayurveda and presented papers as invited speaker at many conferences in both India and abroad. He isthe Principal Investigator of the first National Institutes of Health-supported research project to evaluate Ayurveda outside the United States. He is a member of the Research Advisory Committee, Indian National Science Academy, New Delhi, as well as the Central Council for Indian Medicine, Ministry of Health and Family Welfare, New Delhi. His recent papers include 'Ayurveda and Modern Science: New Sources of Information', at the seminar on 'Indian Traditional Knowledge — History, Influences and New Directions for Natural Science', Bangalore, February 2009, and 'Diagnosis in Ayurveda: Solution oriented troubleshooting', at the 13th International Ayurveda-Symposium 2011, Berstein, Germany, September 2011.

Nisha Money is a US-based preventive medicine physician with a specialisation in global health and integrative medicine. She recently transitioned from active military duty to serve as the Chief Medical Officer for Complementary & Alternative Medicine (CAM)-Integrative Health, in collaboration with the Department of Defense and Veteran Administration for traumatic brain injury and psychological health.

Asha Mukherjee is a Professor at the Department of Philosophy, Visva-Bharati University. Her research interests are Logic, Ethics, Applied Ethics, Analytic Philosophy, Social Philosophy, Epistemology,

Philosophical Logic, Gender Issues, Environmental Ethics and Jaina Philosophy. Her publications include 'Jainism: Its Identity on the Basis of Literature and Philosophy' in *Religion and Literature: Indian Perspective* (Projit Kumar Palited.) (2011), and 'Capability Approach: Theory and Practice' in *Morality and Social Justice* (Abha Singh ed.) (2010).

Piyali Palit retired from the Department of Philosophy, Jadavpur University. She received her Ph.D. in Sanskrit from Rabindra Bharati University, Kolkata. Professor Palit was the Principal Investigator, University Grants Commission Major Research Project on 'Indian Philosophy and Research Methodology'. She has organised a number of training courses and workshops in Manuscriptology, Vaishesika Formal Ontology, Science, Technology and Culture of Ancient India. She was the ICCR Chair Professor in Sanskrit and Indian Philosophy at the School of Indological Studies, Mahatma Gandhi Institute, Mauritius. Her publications include *Basic Principles of Indian Philosophy of Language* (2004).

Nilanjana Sanyal was a Professor at the Department of Psychology, University of Calcutta. Her areas of specialisation are Clinical and Developmental Psychology and Psychodynamics of Relationships. Her publications include 'Aggression Assessment Techniques: A Review', *Journal of Psychometry* 1 (2007), and 'Object-Relations — The Holy Curiosity in Psychoanalysis and Relationships', *Journal of the Asiatic Society of Bangladesh (Hum.)* 52 (1, 2007).

Hartmut Scharfe received his Ph.D. in 1956 from Humboldt University, Berlin. He taught at University of California at Los Angeles for several years and, since his retirement in 1974, continues to be Professor Emeritus of Sanskrit, Pali and Indic Languages in the Department of Asian Languages and Cultures. Internationally known for his path-breaking studies in ancient Indian culture, his major publications include *Grammatical Literature* (1977), *Investigations in Kautalya's Manual of Political Science* (1993), *The State in Indian Tradition* (1989), and *Education in Ancient India* (2002).

V. Sujatha is Associate Professor, Centre for the Study of Social Systems, Jawaharlal Nehru University, New Delhi. She has researched and published in the areas of Pharmaceutical Chemistry and Industrial

Sociology. She is co-editor (with Leena Abraham) of *Medical Pluralism in Contemporary India* (2012) and the author of *Health by the People: Sociology of Medical Lore* (2013).

Anuradha Veeravalli is Assistant Professor, Department of Philosophy, University of Delhi. Her publications include 'Swaraj and Sovereignty', *Economic and Political Weekly*, 46 (5, 2011).

Roger Worthington received his Ph.D. in Philosophy from the State University of New York (Buffalo). He currently holds honorary academic positions at Yale University School of Medicine, USA, and the Faculty of Health Sciences and Medicine at Bond University, Australia. He lives in the UK where he taught medical law and ethics at Keele University School of Medicine. He has a lifelong interest in Indian philosophy and has written two books based on ancient texts. His publications include *Health Policy and Ethics: A Critical Examination of Values from a Global Perspective* (with R. Rohrbaugh) (2011) and an edited volume, *Ethics and Palliative Care: A Case Based Manual* (2005).

O. P. Yadava is CEO and Chief Cardiac Surgeon, National Heart Institute (NHI), New Delhi. He is the editor-in-chief of *Cardiology Today* and *Annals of IMA Academy of Medical Specialities*. He also serves as a member of the editorial board for *Indian Heart Journal*, *Journal of the American Medical Association* (Indian Edition) and *Journal of Cardiovascular Diseases* (Pakistan). His most recent publications include *Electrocardiography — A Revisit* (2007) and an edited volume, *ECAB Clinical Update: Cardiology — Follow-up after Cardiovascular Surgery* (2008).

Index

Milton Keynes UK
Ingram Content Group UK Ltd.
UKHW020000071024
449327UK00031B/2590

9 780367 176914